T0177689

Conscience in Reproductive Health Care

Conscience in Reproductive Health Care

Prioritizing Patient Interests

CAROLYN McLEOD

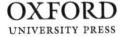

OXFORD

UNIVERSITY PRESS

Great Clarendon Street, Oxford, OX2 6DP,
United Kingdom

Oxford University Press is a department of the University of Oxford.
It furthers the University's objective of excellence in research, scholarship,
and education by publishing worldwide. Oxford is a registered trade mark of
Oxford University Press in the UK and in certain other countries

Published in the United States of America by Oxford University Press
198 Madison Avenue, New York, NY 10016, United States of America

British Library Cataloguing in Publication Data
Data available

Library of Congress Control Number: 2019954806

ISBN 978–0–19–873272–3

Printed and bound in Great Britain by
Clays Ltd, Elcograf S.p.A.

Links to third party websites are provided by Oxford in good faith and
for information only. Oxford disclaims any responsibility for the materials
contained in any third party website referenced in this work.

For Andrew, Abeti, and Mikiyas
And in loving memory of Roderick M. McLeod

Contents

Acknowledgments

I first encountered the phenomenon of conscientious refusal in health care many years ago when I was living and teaching in Tennessee. A health care professional there told me of a patient whose physician conscientiously refused to grant her access to an abortion, and the patient eventually obtained access elsewhere. She was very reluctant to return to her original physician afterwards, because he would know she had had the abortion. At the same time, she had few other options for primary health care. I was both appalled and intrigued by this case. It inspired me to do some writing on conscientious refusals, and I was also encouraged to do so by John Hardwig, a colleague of mine at the time. After some false starts, I came to realize just how morally complex these refusals are. What began as an interest in writing a single paper became a project that I pursued (on and off) for two decades.

The project really got going in 2010 when I created the Conscience Research Group, which was based at my university, Western, and also at Dalhousie University. The members included Françoise Baylis, Jocelyn Downie, Michael Hickson, Daniel Weinstock, Reuven Brandt, Patrick Clipsham, Chlöe Fitzgerald, Lori Kantymir, Jason Marsh, Angel Petropanagos, Margaret O'Brien, Emma Ryman, Jacquelyn Shaw, and Meghan Winsby. I am grateful to them all, but especially to Jocelyn and Françoise, who helped guide the direction of the group. Emma Ryman served as my research assistant for this book. She was incredibly helpful, as shown by the many times I thank her in the text.

Most of the financial support for the Conscience Research Group came from the Canadian Institutes of Health Research (CIHR) grant FRN 102516, "Let Conscience Be Their Guide? Conscientious Refusals in Reproductive Health Care." This funding allowed us to host many educational events, including one where we were educated ourselves by health policy makers from the Colleges of Physicians and Surgeons in Canada. This meeting helped me settle on the position about conscientious refusals that I defend in this book, and so I am particularly thankful for it. I gained new insights not only from the policy makers in attendance, but also from the philosopher Mark Wicclair, who travelled to Canada for this purpose.

My approach to conscientious refusals of prioritizing patient interests is informed by the burgeoning legal scholarship on fiduciary relationships. For guiding me through this literature and answering my questions about it, I am indebted to Dennis Klimchuk, Paul B. Miller, Evan Fox-Decent, Emma Ryman, and Lionel Smith. Workshops I attended on fiduciary relationships were invaluable to me, including "Fiduciaries and Trust," hosted by Matthew Harding at Melbourne Law School in 2018, and "Fiduciary Relationships," which Dennis and I held at Western in 2015. Thanks to everyone who participated in these meetings and for putting up with what were probably naïve questions from me about fiduciaries.

I was fortunate to be able to work with Peter Momtchiloff at Oxford University Press, who was very supportive and patient. I am also grateful for the hard work and professionalism of the production team, including Henry Clarke, Susan Frampton, and Jayashree Thirumaran. Two anonymous reviewers from OUP provided valuable feedback on my manuscript. I thank them both, and especially reviewer A, whose extensive comments helped me to improve the book substantially.

The book was initially conceived during the 2013–14 academic year while I was a Visiting Professor at the Centre for Ethics at the University of Toronto and on sabbatical from Western University. These institutions gave me the space and time I needed to reflect on the work I had already done on conscientious refusals and to map out this book. I was also inspired to take up the challenge of doing a monograph by Shlomi Segall, who was visiting the Centre for Ethics at the same time I was.

Some of the chapters of the book are based on previous publications. Chapters 1 and 2 draw substantially from material in my contribution to *Being Relational*, edited by Jocelyn Downie and Jennifer J. Llewellyn © University of British Columbia Press 2011 (all rights reserved by the Publisher) and from my article, "Harm or Mere Inconvenience? Denying Women Emergency Contraception", *Hypatia*, Volume 25, Issue 1, pp. 11–30, doi: 10.1111/j.1527-2001.2009.01082.x (© Hypatia, Inc. 2010), respectively. Also, Chapter 4 contains material from "Referral in the Wake of Conscientious Objection to Abortion" (*Hypatia* Volume 23, Issue 4, pp. 30–47, doi:10.1111/j.1527-2001.2008.01432.x, © Hypatia, Inc 2008).

I presented work in progress for the book in many venues. I'm especially grateful for the invitations I received to speak from Nir Ben Moshe, Jeanette Kennett, Stephen Clarke, Julian Savulescu, Kate Greasley, Carol Sanger, Sara Goering, Holmer Steinfath, Mark Hall, and Anita Tarzian.

Extended family and friends are a constant source of love and encouragement for me. Special thanks go to my mother, Mary Anne McLeod, and my mother-in-law, Mary Botterell, as well as to Katie McLeod, Andy McLeod, Margaret Whitley, Mark Whitley, Jane Anweiler, Chris Sherrin, Helen Fielding, Jessica Goldberg, Sian Owen, Lorraine Davies, and my friends in Southampton, Ontario.

I would not have the career I have together with the wonderful family life I enjoy were it not for my partner, Andrew Botterell. For years, he supported me in the writing of this book: by commenting on every chapter, often more than once; by lifting my spirits when I got discouraged; and by caring for our children while I worked. I am forever appreciative of him and of our sons, Abeti and Mikiyas. Andrew and I are extremely lucky to be parents of these boys, both of whom are loving, witty, and brave. They, along with Andrew, enrich my life immensely, and so I dedicate this book to the three of them.

My father, Rod McLeod, died just before I made my first submission of the book to the press. I said at his funeral that I would be adrift for a while, but that I would recover because he made me strong. I have recovered, but I still miss him terribly. This book is in memory of him.

Introduction

Conscientious objections by health care professionals to abortion are a pressing global health issue (IWHC 2017; Chavkin et al. 2013). Many countries have in place laws or policies permitting abortion that include clauses providing some protection for conscientious objectors. Although it is difficult to know how often health care professionals exercise the freedom that "conscience clauses" offer them, there is evidence that they are using these policies more and more frequently to avoid having to provide abortions and similar services, such as contraception. For example, a recent report of the International Women's Health Coalition (IWHC)—entitled *Unconscionable*—refers to a "growing global trend" of health care professionals refusing on grounds of conscience "to deliver abortion and other sexual and reproductive health care" (2017, 4).

The moral and political controversy over conscientious refusals in health care is as polarized as the abortion debate itself. While some, including US President Donald Trump,[1] have sought to expand the protections afforded to conscientious objectors, others have argued that conscience clauses should be eliminated altogether (e.g., Schuklenk 2015; Schuklenk and Smalling 2016; Savulescu and Schuklenk 2017). The IWHC, for example, states that health care professionals should not be permitted to "prioritize [their religious or moral beliefs] over their duty to provide services," because such conduct is indeed unconscionable (2017, 4, 5). Rather, according to the IWHC, they should be required to prioritize the interests of patients in receiving services like abortions.

This book defends "the prioritizing approach" to conscientious refusals adopted by the IWHC and others. I contend that conscientious objectors in health care have a moral obligation to prioritize the health care interests of their patients and the public over their own conscience, and that regulations on conscientious refusals should reflect this fact. Although I do not say that all conscientious objection in health care is morally unacceptable, I claim

---

[1] He instituted a "conscience rule" in 2019 that gives broad legal protection for the conscience of health care providers (Sanger-Katz 2019).

Conscience in Reproductive Health Care: Prioritizing Patient Interests. Carolyn McLeod, Oxford University Press (2020).
© Carolyn McLeod.
DOI: 10.1093/oso/9780198732723.001.0001

that most of it should be severely restricted. My goal is to argue for this view, moreover, while acknowledging the moral complexity of conscientious refusals in health care. It is not enough, in my opinion, to say that conscientious objectors should "just do their job or get out of the profession," which is a statement one hears often. Neither is it appropriate to assume that the conscience of health care professionals has no moral value. In arguing that most of the time, conscientious objectors should subordinate their conscience to the health care interests of patients, I am not seeking to downplay the importance that conscience has, or at least can have, in health care settings. To the contrary, I accept that moral conflicts often arise when health care professionals make conscientious objections. I also maintain that these conflicts are resolvable, however, by pointing to the duty health care professionals have to give priority to patients' interests.[2] Hence, the best strategy for dealing with conscientious refusals is the prioritizing approach that I endorse.

The main focus of this book is on *conscience in reproductive health care*, even though conscientious refusals occur in other areas, such as end-of-life care. My arguments extend *mutatis mutandis* to these other refusals, including those that target medical aid in dying (MAID). Like members of the IWHC, however, I am concerned about the prevalence of conscientious refusals in reproductive health care and the extent to which they restrict access to abortion and contraception. As my other work makes clear, I am firmly committed to reproductive autonomy and more specifically, to bodily autonomy in and around pregnancy (see esp. McLeod 2002; Botterell and McLeod 2015). Although my arguments here do not depend on me being correct about the value of reproductive autonomy, my views about it have certainly motivated this project of resisting the widespread use of conscience to deny patients' requests for abortion and contraception.

I will have more to say below about the theme of reproduction in the book. But first let me clarify how I propose to understand the terms "conscientious refusal" and "conscientious objection," which I use interchangeably.

1. Forms of Conscientious Conduct

The literature on conscience in health care refers to different forms of conscientious conduct that health care professionals might engage in. The list

---

[2] On resolvable (or irresolvable) moral conflicts, see Hursthouse (1999).

includes conscientious refusal, conscientious commitment, conscientious compliance, and civil disobedience. I center my attention on the first type of behavior because it has become a substantial barrier to accessing reproductive services like abortions. While I interpret this sort of conduct rather narrowly (more narrowly than the IWHC does, for example),[3] I do so in a way that fits with concerns about patients being denied requests for reproductive health care. With that in mind, let me describe what I see as the four main features of *conscientious refusals*. I will explain along the way what is distinctive about this form of conduct compared to other forms that emanate from conscience.

First and perhaps most obvious, conscientious refusals involve refusing to behave in a way that conflicts with one's conscience. The conduct issues from conscience, rather than simply being careful or meticulous (which is one way to interpret "conscientious"). In addition, conscience itself has a moral dimension to it (see Chapter 1); it is informed by one's secular or religious moral values. Conscientious refusal is therefore a type of moral behavior. The fact that it stems from conscience, and therefore from one's moral values, is a quality it shares with other forms of conscientious conduct, such as conscientious compliance or commitment.

Second, with conscientious refusal, one must refuse to do something (or object to something), and for health care professionals that "something" is the standard of care. Conscientious objectors in health care refuse to offer services that make up this standard, which they are expected to provide given their specialty. Such services must be legally required or permitted and deemed by the objector's health professional association to be central to good health care. I call them "standard services." To illustrate, where health care professionals conscientiously refuse to perform abortions, the standard of care for patients who face an unwanted pregnancy and who conscientiously decide in favor of an abortion is to have access to one. The expectation is that all health care professionals who have a certain specialty or specialties, or who work in certain contexts (e.g., a reproductive health care clinic), will provide this care. What conscience clauses do, where they exist, is remove or relax this requirement for conscientious objectors. These professionals issue their refusals and then the clauses protect their behavior. In this way,

---

[3] For them, conscientious objection in health care involves the refusal to provide a service that conflicts with one's "religious, ethical, or other beliefs" (2017, 8). In my view, the refusal must stem from (secular or religious) moral beliefs and must also normally be done in response to a request by a patient for the offending service.

conscientious objection—again, objecting on grounds of conscience to the expectation that one will offer standard services—can be legally or professionally permissible.

Third, the express goal of a conscientious objection is normally to seek protection for one's conscience, rather than to effect change in law or policy. Although conscientious objectors may sincerely hope that the health laws or policies they are resisting will be abandoned,[4] this result is not their focus when they make their refusals, which—to be clear—they do primarily in the presence of patients and in the relative privacy of their clinical practice. If they wanted to do more than practice health care in accordance with their conscience, then they would likely make their objections more public than they tend to do. These points reveal how conscientious refusal differs from *civil disobedience*, where the latter is "a public, non-violent and conscientious breach of law undertaken with the aim of bringing about a change in laws or government policies" (Brownlee 2013, citing Rawls 1971). Civilly disobedient actors openly violate the law with an awareness and willing acceptance of the legal consequences of their actions. By contrast, conscientious objectors may not be breaking any law, for there could be a conscience clause in place that legally protects their behavior. They are also usually determined to receive protection for their conscience. Though not my focus in this book, civil disobedience in health care is a real and important phenomenon. The Canadian physician, Henry Morgentaler, for example, chose this method of action to support his stand in favor of abortion access. Morgentaler openly defied Canada's restrictive abortion law, which was struck down as a direct result of his conscientious action and of legal appeals he made of his own convictions under the law (Marshall and McLaren 2013; Dickens 2008). He achieved what he set out to do, which was primarily to bring about legal reform rather than to safeguard his conscience. The latter is a feature of conscientious refusals, but not of civil disobedience.[5]

Fourth and finally, conscientious refusals are commonly a response to a request by a patient for a standard service. The refusals do more than merely target what (objectors believe) is a problematic standard of care. Because objectors are refusing to do what patients want from them, the patients must by hypothesis disagree with the refusal. The objector and the patient are

---

[4] I owe this point to an anonymous reviewer of the OUP.

[5] Features like the first three I've discussed—conscientious refusals are motivated by conscience, they are reactions against an external standard imposed on the objector, and they aim at protecting conscience—are common to all conscientious refusals, including those that occur in domains other than health care.

therefore in conflict with one another. They are the main parties to conflicts of conscience that occur when health care professionals conscientious refuse to provide standard services.[6]

In contrast, with other types of conscientious conduct, including conscientious commitment and compliance, the patient normally agrees with what the objector does. *Conscientious commitment*, which Bernard Dickens and Rebecca Cook describe as "the reverse of conscientious objection" (2011), involves not a refusal but rather a commitment to provide services on grounds of conscience. In such cases, the services are not standard since they are prohibited by law or policy (often hospital policy). The health care professional also usually offers them with the patient's consent. To illustrate, Morgentaler engaged in this form of action as well as in civil disobedience (which I interpret as a kind of conscientious commitment). He was conscientiously committed to providing patients with abortion access, which one could presumably do without publicly striving to dismantle laws or policies that oppose such access. Since Morgentaler also did the latter, his conduct counts in my books as civil disobedience *and* as conscientious commitment.

Similarly, with *conscientious compliance*, the patient usually authorizes or approves of the health care professional's conscientious action (or would do so if the action were made transparent to the patient). Conscientiously compliant professionals abide by laws or policies that they deem to be unjust; yet they do so in a way that conforms as much as possible to their conscience (Buchbinder et al. 2016). The main example in the literature involves "Women's Right To Know" (WRTK) laws, which exist in many US states and which mandate certain kinds of counseling before an abortion can be performed. Some physicians believe—rightly, I think—that the "counseling" includes information that is either medically irrelevant or not supported by the available medical evidence, and that is designed simply to make patients question their abortion decisions (see Gold and Nash 2007; Rodrigues 2014).[7] By engaging in conscientious compliance with these laws, physicians provide the mandated information in a way that should make it clear to the patient that they believe the information is unnecessary

---

[6] That is not to say there are no other parties to these conflicts, including health policy-makers and colleagues of conscientious objectors who have to do the work that the objectors refuse to do.

[7] It can involve showing the patient the fetus on an ultrasound, descriptions of the fetus at different stages of development, and information about risks of an abortion for which there is no medical evidence (e.g., the procedure could cause breast cancer; Gold and Nash 2007).

or misleading. Since these physicians are not refusing to provide a mandated service (an informational one), they are not, strictly speaking, conscientiously refusing. Neither are they engaging in conscientious commitment or civil disobedience. Instead, they are performing a unique kind of conscientious action.

To be clear, the final feature of conscientious refusals—that they involve a negative response to a request by a patient and therefore give rise to a conflict with the patient—is common to this form of conduct, but is not necessary for it, in my view. Health care professionals might refuse on grounds of conscience to comply, rather than choose conscientiously to comply, with something like a WRTK law. And they could do so with the consent of their patients. We would probably describe such conduct as a conscientious refusal even though it does not involve a conflict with a patient. Labeling it this way, moreover, is perfectly consistent with my theory, because I accept that there can be conscientious refusals that are made on behalf of patients, that is, with their consent. (I return to this issue in Chapter 5.)

The fact that the patient does not authorize the health care professional's action is nevertheless unique to most conscientious refusals. It is also morally salient. One might think that the strong stand I take against these refusals carries over to all other forms of conscientious conduct (e.g., conscientious commitment), making me as opposed to them as I am to conscientious refusals (typical ones at least). This result would be worrisome, because it would mean that I would be dedicated to opposing the conscientious commitment of health care professionals to provide abortions, or similar services, in jurisdictions where they are illegal. The fact that such action would be performed with the patient's consent, however, is morally significant in my view—so much so that the action can indeed be morally permissible.[8] Although I reserve a full discussion of this topic for another time, I raise it here to forestall what is an important objection to the kind of position I take on conscientious refusals.

To summarize, conscientious refusals are refusals made by health care professionals, on grounds of conscience, to patients' requests for services that make up the standard of care the professionals are meant to provide to patients, given their specialty or the context in which they work. As a result,

---

[8] I do suggest briefly why or when it would be permissible in Chapter 5. To be clear, my view is that where abortion is illegal, health care professionals should engage in civil disobedience and perform abortions, depending on the likely consequences of that action for themselves or others. They should model their behavior, in other words, after that of Henry Morgentaler.

such conduct puts health care professionals in conflict with patients. Most conscientious refusals in health care fit this description, including those that the IWHC and similar groups oppose. Throughout the book, my attention centers on this sort of conduct rather than on unusual forms of conscientious refusal (i.e., where the patient consents to the refusal) or on entirely different forms of conscientious action, such as conscientious compliance or commitment.

2. Power, Priority, and Procreation

Conscience and conscientious refusals are central themes of this book. But so are power, priority, and procreation. I've already indicated why procreation is important, and I will expand further on that explanation here. "Priority" refers to my prioritizing approach. And lastly, there is power: specifically, the power wielded by conscientious objectors. Let me begin by discussing it.

Overall, the book highlights the power of conscientious objectors in health care. My focus is on objectors who count as health care professionals (not as health care staff who are not professionals, or as health care institutions).[9] I also home in on professionals who are meant to control access to health care services and who therefore play a *gatekeeping* role.[10] (Here and throughout, "health care professional" refers to professionals of this type.) The relevant professionals when it comes to access to abortions or contraception are physicians and pharmacists, and sometimes also nurse practitioners or midwives. In their roles as health care professionals and gatekeepers, these people have power. While some of them have the social power (i.e., the prestige and the high income) that accompanies being a

[9] These individuals or entities have objected on grounds of conscience to providing, or participating in the provision, of standard services. (On objections by health care institutions, see Wicclair 2011, Chapter 4; and Shadd and Shadd 2017.) They sometimes—though relatively rarely—receive legal protection for these claims. For example, President Trump's "conscience rule" extends to health care workers who are not professionals (see note 1). I concentrate neither on these workers nor on health care institutions, because I assume that any conscience protection they are owed could not be greater than what is owed to health care professionals, which in my view is very little.

[10] I do that even though the conscientious objections of health care professionals who are not gatekeepers can be very disruptive. For example, between 1988 and 1990, "it was nearly impossible for a woman to obtain a second trimester abortion for social reasons in an SA [South Australia] hospital...The cause...was the mass refusal by SA nurses, on grounds of conscience, to participate in [these] abortions" (Cannold 1994, 80).

certain kind of health care professional, particularly a physician, all of them have power as *fiduciaries* for their patients and for the public they serve: power in the form of discretionary authority to make decisions that affect important interests of patients and the public (see Chapters 5 and 6). Physicians especially tend to be perceived as fiduciaries for their patients. The fact that they have power in this role is poorly understood in bioethics, however, and is entirely absent from bioethical discussion about conscientious refusals. This, I believe, is an important oversight. Drawing from the legal literature on fiduciaries, I explain that to be a fiduciary is to have a special kind of power, one that resides in those who act as gatekeepers to health care services. I claim that with this power comes great responsibility,[11] enough to severely limit the protection that objectors are morally owed for their conscience.

My central thesis in this book is that due to their fiduciary role, health care professionals must prioritize the health care interests of patients over their interest in acting on their conscience. Although both parties' interests tend to be morally substantial, the interests of patients should take priority because of the fiduciary duties that conscientious objectors owe to patients. Accommodation for conscientious objectors is therefore warranted only when it would pose no threat to patients' health care interests. It follows that the primary objective in regulating these refusals should be to protect patients, not health care professionals. I focus on conscientious objections to abortion or contraception and argue that in all likelihood, protection for them sets patients' health interests back, even in cases where the patients could go to another professional nearby to obtain the service they seek. Conscience protection in these cases is therefore morally problematic. I argue in this way for what I've called "the prioritizing approach" to conscientious refusals in reproductive health care.[12]

An alternative to prioritizing patients' interests is to strike a compromise between the objectors and the patients. This approach is popular among bioethicists,[13] some of whom describe it in terms of a balancing of interests. I argue that we should reject this alternative for two reasons: first, in many

---

[11] Here, I am paraphrasing Uncle Ben from the Spiderman series (Ziskin and Bruce 2002).

[12] I call it *the* prioritizing approach rather than *a* prioritizing approach, because I believe that the alternative of prioritizing the interests of conscientious objectors over those of patients is a nonstarter, morally speaking. See Chapter 5.

[13] For example, it's the approach taken by Mark Wicclair and Holly Fernandez Lynch, both of whom have given book-length treatments to conscientious refusals (Wicclair 2011; Lynch 2008).

cases of conscientious refusal, compromise is unrealistic; and second, this strategy is not compatible with health care professionals putting their patients' interests ahead of their own interests. I conclude, therefore, that the compromise approach is morally unsound. (I also use the term "compromise" rather than "balancing" to describe it throughout, because in my view, compromise and balancing are not the same thing. Balancing competing interests involves weighing them to decide which interest might prevail, or to determine how to accommodate both interests so that one fully appreciates their value. By contrast, devising a compromise between parties with conflicting interests involves identifying reasons each party has to accept a position that promotes each of their interests to some extent. I employ this theory about the nature of compromise in my critique of the compromise approach. I also assume that what defenders of it actually prefer is compromise rather than balancing.)

One final theme of the book is procreation. Throughout, my discussion centers on typical conscientious refusals in reproductive health care, which are refusals that target requests by patients for a service that, in the mind of the objector, threatens unborn life. I call these simply "typical refusals." The relevant services include abortion; oral contraception of the kind that some believe can interfere with the implantation of an embryo, thereby causing its death (and making the method deserving of the label, "abortifacient"); and in vitro fertilization, which usually involves the destruction of unusable or unused embryos. I mention IVF even though conscientious refusals to perform IVF out of concern for the deaths of human embryos are not typical, since health care professionals who take the time to learn IVF techniques are not people who would be inclined to turn down all requests for IVF. What is more typical of health care professionals who are concerned with saving unborn lives are refusals to refer patients for IVF to fertility specialists. Such conduct does qualify as a typical refusal, and much of what I say is directly relevant to it, although for reasons I've already mentioned, I pay particular attention to refusals to provide abortions and contraception. Let me say more about why I focus on these services.

First, conscientious objection to these basic forms of reproductive health care is prevalent worldwide, probably more so than any other type of conscientious refusal;[14] and this fact allows me to concentrate on them while

---

[14] For example, conscientious objection to MAID by those who specialize in end-of-life care is surely not as common as refusals to perform abortions, mainly because abortion is legal in many more places than MAID is.

still making general claims about how all refusals should be regulated. To explain, since conscientious objections to abortion and contraception are relatively common, any general policy on conscientious objection should be consistent with the ethics of these particular refusals. I refer to both specific and general policies on conscientious refusals: that is, ones that are specific to a particular type of refusal—an example being a conscience clause on abortion—and ones that are general in the sense that they are meant to apply to all types of refusals. An example of the latter is a policy on (all) conscientious refusals of a regulating body such as a College of Physicians and Surgeons in Canada.[15] I claim that the general policies should resemble the specific ones that are designed for typical refusals (e.g., to perform abortions), if only because these refusals are very common.

Second, conscientious refusals to provide abortions or contraception restrict the right to *not* reproduce, which I believe is extremely important, especially for patients who have the capacity to become pregnant. Of course, conscientious refusals can occur in the realm of medically assisted reproduction and can infringe on patients' right *to* reproduce (an example being a refusal to perform egg freezing as insurance against age-related infertility where this service has become standard; see Harwood 2009). Elsewhere I've expressed skepticism about whether the right to reproduce even exists, however (see Botterell and McLeod 2015). This fact explains why I am less concerned about the barriers that conscientious objections pose to assisted reproduction compared to techniques that are designed to prevent reproduction (which is not to say, of course, that I have no concern for the former).

Third, the prioritizing approach is more controversial when it is applied to refusals to provide abortions and contraception, compared to other conscientious refusals.[16] Commentators sometimes say that these typical refusals merely inconvenience patients rather than harm them, especially if the patients can easily go somewhere else to obtain the services they seek (see, e.g., Fenton and Lomasky 2005). By contrast, remarks of this kind are missing from discussions about other kinds of refusals, including those that focus on MAID. People tend not to think—for good reason, in my view—that it is

---

[15] See, e.g., the College of Physicians and Surgeons of Ontario's policy #2-15, "Professional Obligations and Human Rights"—particularly "B) Conscience or Religious Beliefs"—at http://www.cpso.on.ca/policies-publications/policy/professional-obligations-and-human-rights (retrieved May 19, 2019).

[16] The same is true of the compromise approach, for if patients are merely inconvenienced by refusals to provide abortions or contraception, then why should objectors agree to compromise with them?

ever a mere inconvenience to be conscientiously denied MAID, despite qualifying for it. Exactly why there is this difference in debates about access to MAID versus access to abortion or contraception is no doubt complex.[17] Nevertheless, the fact that the difference exists means that taking the prioritizing approach to conscientious objections to abortion and contraception is particularly controversial. The lesson we are supposed to take from the claim that this conduct merely inconveniences patients is that it is not very serious; its impact on patients does not warrant placing restrictions on the conscience of health care professionals. I argue that this view is deeply mistaken.

My main concern in the book is therefore with typical refusals, especially those that are directed toward patients' requests for abortion or contraception. But let me comment briefly on another type of refusal and also on my use of the term "patient." Some conscientious refusals target people rather than health care services. A prominent example in the realm of reproductive health care is the refusal to provide LGBTQ+ people with access to medically assisted reproduction (Merritt 2008; Robinson 1997). Since most bioethicists believe—correctly, in my opinion—that conscientious objections amounting to invidious discrimination are morally out of bounds, I do not focus on these objections,[18] although my arguments certainly extend to them, as they do to most other conscientious refusals in health care.

Related to my blanket opposition to discriminatory refusals and refusals to provide LGBTQ+ people with reproductive health care is my use of the term "patients" rather than "women" (or "girls") to refer to those whose requests for abortion or contraception are denied. I deliberately employ this terminology because not all of these patients will identify, or be identified, as women; for example, some will be non-binary individuals, and some will be trans men who engage in same-sex sexual activity and have the capacity to become pregnant.[19] As a feminist ethicist, I am deeply concerned about

---

[17] The explanation may have to do with differences in how people generally obtain these services (abortion and contraception versus MAID), how easy it is to obtain them from non-objecting health care professionals, and whether the public genuinely believes that people have a right to them. Oppressive stereotypes that make people think negatively about patients who seek out an abortion or emergency contraception can certainly influence public opinion about whether patients ultimately have a right to these services. (For a discussion about relevant stereotypes, see Chapters 2 and 3.)

[18] For similar reasons, I also do not discuss in depth refusals to provide care in emergencies or to inform patients about their health care options.

[19] I also avoid using the adjective "female" to refer to patients who have this capacity (i.e., to become pregnant) because not all of them are female; some, rather, are intersex individuals (see Fausto-Sterling 2000).

the oppression not only of women, but also of LGBTQ+ people who are not women. What is more, I am committed to a world in which gender becomes increasingly fluid and less morally significant than it currently is for most people. Referring to the relevant patients as simply "patients" is consistent with this ideal but also with the fact that, again, not all patients seeking the services I'm concerned with are women. Where it is important, I do discuss how patients are or can be oppressed in society (e.g., as women), rather than assume that the ideal world I cherish already exists. I also use the term "patient" to refer to actual or prospective patients, unless I specify one over the other.[20]

To sum up, along with my terminological point about "patients," this section has been devoted to explaining how and why I concentrate on conscientious refusals that concern *procreation* (or more accurately the avoidance of it), the general approach I take to these refusals (one that gives *priority* to patients' interests), and how I justify this approach by appealing to the *power* that health care professionals have as fiduciaries.

3. Structure

Let me turn lastly to the overall shape of the book. There are two main parts to it. The first describes what is at stake for the main parties to the conflict generated by a typical conscientious refusal—the objector and the patient—while the second part defends the prioritizing approach to typical refusals and offers suggestions about how to regulate such conduct by health care professionals. There are six chapters in total: three in each part of the book. Together, they lead to the conclusion that patient interests should be prioritized over objectors' interests. The chapters also stand alone, however, so that readers who have specific questions about the morality of conscientious objection could concentrate on the chapters that most interest them.

Part I looks at why it is important to value conscience in health care, what health care professionals might lose if we did not protect their conscientious conduct, and the threats that typical conscientious refusals pose to patients. I contend in Chapter 1 that conscience has value, generally speaking, in health care, although not because it leads health care professionals on the path to moral righteousness or truth, as some would have it. Rather, it can

---

[20] Patients also needn't be passive recipients of medical advice or treatment, but rather can be empowered to direct their own health care. It is customary in feminist bioethics to assume the term "patient" has this meaning, and I follow this custom.

allow health care professionals to have integrity, which itself has personal and social value. The claim that conscience promotes integrity is common in bioethics, although I interpret "integrity" differently than most bioethicists do (e.g., Blustein 1993; Childress 1979; Benjamin 1995; Wicclair 2000, 2011). Overall, I develop a novel theory about the nature and value of conscience, and also respond to questions like the following: Would anything of value really be lost if we were to prohibit conscientious refusals in health care? and Should we not just say to conscientious objectors, "park your conscience at the door"? While my answer to the first question is yes, my answer to the second is that such statements are misguided and insensitive. In short, they fail to grapple with the moral complexity of conscientious refusals in health care.

With respect to patients, I argue that rather than merely inconvenience those who could get the relevant services nearby, it is likely that typical refusals harm them. Since good empirical evidence is lacking about the impact of such conduct on patients, I have to speculate about its impact, which I do based on various factors, including the power dynamic between health care professionals and patients, and the well-documented stigma that patients experience when they request services like abortions. I argue that in light of these factors, typical refusals probably do cause harm and do so, in particular, by threatening the moral identity of patients (as good or fine people), their sense of security (in being able to control what happens to their body), or their reproductive autonomy. These claims appear in Chapter 2, while Chapter 3 focuses on the harm that conscientious refusals cause when they diminish the trust that patients have in health care professionals and professions. I argue that damage to trust from typical refusals is very likely to occur, because of the nature of these refusals as well as the nature of trust. The main question I respond to in these chapters is: Don't typical refusals just inconvenience patients rather than harm them? My answer is a firm no.

The conclusion to Part I is that important interests are at stake in regulating typical refusals in reproductive health care, and that this is true for both conscientious objectors and patients. One might think, then, that devising a compromise between the parties would be the best way to deal with these conflicts. In Part II, I reject this approach, however, and argue instead in favor of the approach that prioritizes patient interests. My critique of the compromise approach appears in Chapter 4, where I maintain that developing a good compromise—even a true (i.e., genuine) one—is unlikely to happen for typical refusals (again, those where the objector seeks to protect the life of "the unborn"). The discussion in this chapter focuses on what has been called the "conventional compromise," which is that conscientious objectors can refuse to provide the service that morally offends them so long as they give a proper referral for it: that is, a referral to a colleague who is willing and able to provide the relevant service. In answer to the question, Does the policy of requiring proper referrals amount to a true compromise?, I say no, at least not for many typical objectors. The search for a good compromise for these objectors will be in vain, I argue. We should therefore abandon the compromise approach to regulating typical refusals specifically, as well as all refusals generally, because of how common the typical ones are.

A further criticism I make of employing the strategy of compromise is that it represents the interests of objectors and patients as being on par with one another, thereby ignoring the professional role and duties of the objector. In Chapters 5 and 6, I develop the argument that health care professionals who are charged with controlling access to health care services should be viewed as fiduciaries for their patients and for the public. These chapters bring a burgeoning legal literature on fiduciaries to bear on the bioethical issue of conscientious objection. Chapter 5 discusses cases where the request for the offending service comes from a current patient, someone with whom the objector is in an established (fiduciary) relationship. By contrast, Chapter 6 centers on cases where the request comes from a prospective patient, someone who is a member of the public that the objector is licensed to serve.

The claims I make in Chapter 5 are threefold: that health care professionals are fiduciaries (at least while serving in their gatekeeping role); that they therefore have a fiduciary duty of loyalty to their patients; and that this duty prohibits them from making typical objections because doing so jeopardizes the health interests of their patients. I explain why this argument works even though typical objectors tend to view the fetus or embryo whose life is at risk as their second patient. In general, Chapter 5 answers the following: What does the widely recognized duty of health care professionals to give primacy to their patients' interests imply about typical refusals? What type of duty is this [answer: fiduciary] and how should these refusals be regulated because of it? In responding to the question about regulation, I argue that severe restrictions are in order. At the same time, I claim that making a proper referral rather than providing the offending service oneself can be a morally appropriate option for a conscientious objector. That is true because sometimes the most loyal thing one can do for one's patients is to refer them to someone else, because of how vehemently one objects to the service they have requested.

Chapter 6 focuses on a duty—endorsed by licensing bodies and health professional organizations—that health care professionals have to the public to promote public health, and more narrowly, to foster equitable access to health care.[21] I argue that this duty is a type of fiduciary duty, though a different type than the one health care professionals have in their relationships with current patients. The duty to the public demands the professional's fidelity not to individual people, but to abstract purposes, which is the case for many fiduciaries of the public (e.g., CEOs of government corporations; Miller and Gold 2015). I highlight the moral requirement that health care professionals be loyal to the purposes of furthering equitable access and public health, which they can achieve only by prioritizing the interests of prospective patients in gaining access to care over their personal interests. At the same time, they can satisfy this requirement by giving proper referrals, or even by being shielded (e.g., by sympathetic employers or colleagues) from encountering requests by prospective patients that morally offend them. I explain throughout why these claims are true for typical refusals, and in doing so answer the question: Should policy restrictions on these refusals be as strict when the person requesting care is not the objector's own patient? My answer is no, although I do say that serious restrictions should be placed on this behavior.

The central conclusion of Part II is that the prioritizing approach to regulating typical refusals is morally justified. That is true regardless of whether the patient could access the relevant service somewhere else close by and of whether the refusals occur inside or outside of patient–health care professional relationships. By prioritizing the interests of patients and the public over the conscience of health care professionals, we recognize the fiduciary relationships that health care professionals have with these parties and acknowledge the power they have over them as a result.

I began this introduction with a discussion about what the IWHC calls the "growing global trend" of health care professionals conscientiously objecting to performing abortions and similar reproductive services, thereby restricting access to them. This book opposes this type of conscientious conduct by health care professionals and the policies that allow for it. I propose instead that we have policies requiring health care professionals to prioritize patients' interests in receiving standard services—particularly abortions and contraception—over their own interest in abiding by their conscience. Being content with more permissive policies on conscientious refusals would be unconscionable, in my view.

---

[21] Chapter 6 also includes a complete summary of my views about conscientious objections: those that occur inside and outside of patient–health care professional relationships.

PART I
WHAT'S AT STAKE

1

The Value of Conscience

Should we be concerned with protecting the conscience of health care professionals? What is at stake in *not* offering them this protection? These questions, though specific to the health care context, concern the value, generally speaking, of being able to act with a conscience. If there was no value to acting in this way, then there would nothing important at stake in preventing health care professionals from doing so. What is more, conscientious refusals would pose no moral problem, and so having a sustained moral discussion about them would be pointless. This view, though compelling to some perhaps, is not the one I support in this chapter. Instead, I argue that acting with a conscience can have value, and I assume this value is manifest in many cases of conscientious refusal in health care, including typical cases in reproductive health care (i.e., those in which the objector is concerned with preserving the lives of embryos and fetuses). There is often (not always) something important at stake in denying conscientious objectors protection for their conscience.

Many bioethicists claim, without qualification, that there is value in allowing health care professionals to act on their conscience, and that this value lies in supporting their *moral integrity*. On this view, having a conscience involves being compelled to act in accordance with one's own secular or religious moral values, which furthers one's moral integrity. The value of conscience just is the value of this integrity. Although it may seem odd to point to a different quality—integrity—to describe the value of conscience, I have sympathy for this view and defend a version of it here. I simply understand "integrity" differently than other bioethicists who have drawn this connection between conscience and integrity.

To be clear, bioethicists who have the sort of view just described do not all interpret "integrity" in the same way. Most of them understand it in terms of having an integrated self or inner psychological unity, whereas at least one of them—Mark Wicclair—defines integrity in terms of acting in accordance with commitments that define us (i.e., that are "identity-conferring";

Conscience in Reproductive Health Care: Prioritizing Patient Interests. Carolyn McLeod, Oxford University Press (2020).
© Carolyn McLeod.
DOI: 10.1093/oso/9780198732723.001.0001

McFall 1987).[1] I limit my attention mostly to the former view—what I call the "Unity View"—because it provides a good foil for my own theory about conscience and moral integrity, and because it is the most common and most detailed theory of its kind in bioethics.[2] Advocates of the Unity View include James Childress (1979; 1997), Jeffrey Blustein (1993), Martin Benjamin (1995), and Daniel Sulmasy (2008).

In what follows, I clarify the Unity View, indicate why I believe it is flawed, and sketch a positive alternative to it. My engagement with the Unity View appears in the first part of the chapter. There, I argue that conscience often fails to promote inner unity, regardless of the degree of inner unity we have in mind. To the contrary, acting with a conscience can leave people seriously divided rather than unified. In the second (and final) part, I claim that a better view about conscience says that having a conscience encourages us to take our moral values seriously and to revise our values when they do not fit with what we actively endorse. Once we embrace the revised values, they will influence our conscience, making it dynamic rather than fixed. Although not every conscience will be dynamic in this way, a conscience that has significant value will have this quality and in turn will promote our moral integrity, understood in terms not of moral unity but of acting on our best moral judgment (Calhoun 1995). There are important social dimensions to conscience, on this view: to its value, which is partly social, and to the conditions necessary for having a conscience of value.[3] My

---

[1] The former is identical to what Cheshire Calhoun calls the "integrated-self picture of integrity" (1995, 236–41), and to what I would call simply the "unity" picture. Calhoun distinguishes this view about integrity from what she names the "identity" view, according to which integrity involves acting in accordance with commitments that define us (McFall 1987; Calhoun 1995, 241–6). In his most recent work on conscientious objection in health care, Wicclair clarifies that he has an identity view of integrity (2017), whereas I had assumed in an earlier version of this chapter (2012) that he had a unity view. I made this assumption because Wicclair had favorably cited other bioethicists who hold this view (2000, note 25), and also because the two views overlap significantly with one another. Similarities between them are evident in Calhoun's work (1995) and are also highlighted in my discussion below.

[2] For what it's worth, I do think that Wicclair's view about conscience is less developed than the Unity View. To be sure, Wicclair goes a long way toward defending the identity conception of integrity (2017), but he says relatively little about how or why *conscience* protects integrity, so understood. How does this view about conscience fit with the language we tend to associate with conscience: for example, that a good conscience is "clean" and "easy," rather than "troubled" or "uneasy"? Wicclair may very well have good answers to this question, but unlike say Childress and Blustein, he doesn't provide them.

[3] A previous version of this chapter appeared in a book on relational theory, where I referred to my view as "relational" (2012). Like feminists who describe autonomy as relational (see, e.g., Mackenzie and Stoljar 2000, Sherwin 1998, McLeod 2002), I defined conscience as relational. Since not all readers will be familiar with relational theory, however, which is complicated, I will not use the term "relational" here.

argument highlights the social elements of conscience that concern oppression and privilege. So in the end, my view is best described as the "Socio-political, Dynamic View" of conscience, although for simplicity, I call it the "Dynamic View." My contention is that *it* does a better job than the Unity View of explaining what it means to have a conscience, why having a conscience can be valuable, and when and how we ought to value conscience in health care.

Let me make one note of caution before continuing. What is most important for my project in this book is that conscience has (or at least can have) value. For again, if conscience has no value, then the problem of conscientious refusals in health care vanishes; health care professionals should not be afforded any conscience protection if having a conscience is valueless. The remainder of this book hinges on me being correct not so much about why conscience can have value, but about conscience having value at all, in enough cases of conscientious refusal that we should care about the issue of conscience protection for health care professionals. At the same time, readers should understand why I believe that conscience can have substantial value, and also why there is a good alternative to the Unity View. I assume I am not alone in being skeptical of it.

1. Analyzing the Unity View

1.1 The View in a Nutshell

In answer to the general question of why we ought to take conscientious refusals seriously, the Unity View says that a person's integrity is at stake. Blustein writes, for example, that it "is in terms of [a] moral interest in personal integrity that I will understand the significance of appeals to conscience" (1993, 297). Advocates of Unity View variously associate integrity with *wholeness* (Benjamin 1995, 470; Childress 1979, 322; Blustein 1993, 300; Sulmasy 2008, 138), *consistency* (Childress 1979, 321),[4] *inner harmony* (Blustein1993, 298; Childress 1979, 321), *personal integration* (Blustein 1993, 297), and *unity* (Benjamin 1995, 470)—hence, the "Unity" View. Clearly,

---

[4] For example, Childress claims that the slogan, "Let your conscience be your guide," translates into "Let there be consistency and harmony between belief and action under the threat that inconsistency will undermine integrity and occasion a bad conscience" (1979, 321).

their concern is with personal integrity understood in terms of inner unity.[5] (In what follows, "integrity" refers to inner unity, unless noted otherwise.)

According to the Unity View, our conscience has a specific focus: the impact on the self of violating our deep moral commitments.[6] The view is that such conduct would bring about guilt, shame, or self-betrayal that aches so much, we would be unable to live with ourselves. Negative moral emotions like these signal a rupture in the self, between one's actions or thoughts and one's moral values. In other words, they reveal a lack of integrity. On the Unity View, to have a conscience is to be internally warned or reminded of this consequence should one behave in a certain way, and to be reluctant to simply live with this consequence rather than try to prevent or remove it.[7] As this brief summary suggests, there are two dimensions to having a conscience on the Unity View: 1) being alert to signs of discord between our actions or thoughts and our deep moral commitments; and 2) being inclined to assuage the discord. The "voice" of conscience is captured by this alertness and this inclination; our conscience "speaks" to us when we are attentive to and prepared to eliminate inner moral discord.[8]

The idea that we act on our conscience to spare ourselves of inner moral conflict might seem completely wrongheaded. Surely what we seek to do instead is what is morally right, or more weakly, what is not morally wrong.[9] Advocates of the Unity View insist, however, that with conscience, the "focus is not so much on the...rightness or wrongness of a particular act as on the consequences for the self of one's performing it" (Benjamin 1995, 470). And indeed, they have strong reasons for doing so. For example, they explain that making an appeal to conscience to avoid having to perform an action Y is different from expressing or acting in accordance with one's

---

[5] Many feminist philosophers have challenged this way of understanding integrity; see, e.g., Davion (1991), Walker (1998), and Calhoun (1995). I do not do so here in any detail, since my purpose is to understand conscience not integrity, although do see McLeod (2004; 2005).

[6] Many or all of these commitments may be identity-conferring. But the Unity View demands that we live up to them not to preserve our identity so much as to achieve inner unity. Hence, the View interprets "integrity" in terms of unity, not identity. See note 1.

[7] Advocates of the Unity View accept that conscience can operate prospectively—warning us of inner disunity if we behave badly—or retrospectively—highlighting the inner disunity we suffer after having behaved badly (see, e.g., Benjamin 1995, 470).

[8] The Unity View says that we must *heed* our conscience, of course, if we are to have inner unity: a conscience that promotes inner unity is a *good* conscience. But this view also implies that most of us *will* heed our conscience most of the time because it will threaten us with disunity so severe that we will be unable to get on with our lives. For this reason and for brevity's sake, I sometimes refer to what promotes inner unity on the Unity View as simply "conscience" or "having a conscience."

[9] This sort of objection comes from an anonymous reviewer for OUP.

judgment that Y is morally wrong. As Blustein notes (1993, 294), if there were no difference between the two, then making an appeal to conscience, after insisting that Y is wrong, would be redundant. Most of us would agree, however, that the appeal is not redundant, and that must be because it does more than simply express our judgment that Y is wrong. What it says in addition, according to the Unity View, is that our integrity is at stake.

The following are further reasons provided in support of the Unity View and the attention it gives to what we personally endure if we act badly. First, the "dramatic language" that often accompanies an appeal to conscience reveals that what conscience does is protect our integrity (Childress 1997, 404; Benjamin 1995, 470). Examples include "I wouldn't be able to live with myself if I did that"; "I wouldn't be able to sleep at night"; or "I would hate myself." People say such things when they imagine having to violate a commitment that they hold dear, and when they believe the violation would make them feel so alienated from themselves, so de-stabilized, that soldiering on would be difficult, if not impossible. The self-betrayal and subsequent loss of self-respect, together with feelings of shame or guilt, would be unbearable to them. Ultimately, they would lose integrity.

Second, conscience imposes sanctions on our own behavior and not on the behavior of others. It makes no sense to claim, "My conscience says . . . *you* ought to do this or ought not to have done that" (Ryle 1940, 31; cited in Benjamin 1995, 470). The focus on what "I" ought to do, or not do, suggests a concern for me—for my self, and perhaps for my integrity—rather than simply a concern for what is morally right.

Third, and finally, a good conscience is normally described as "quiet," "clean," and "easy," whereas a bad conscience is "troubled" or "uneasy" (Childress 1979, 318; Childress 2006). When we have a good conscience, we are at peace; we are right with ourselves. In other words, we feel whole.

The above reasons show why the Unity View of conscience should be taken seriously. It makes sense of common intuitions about conscience and the role that conscience plays in our moral and psychological lives. Still, I think this view is inadequate as an account of the nature and value of conscience. Let me explain why after first clarifying further aspects of it.[10]

---

[10] One aspect I will leave out of the body of the chapter is that having a conscience is not the same as being morally unified; rather, it serves to preserve or foster this unity. Having a conscience may be necessary for moral unity, but it could not be sufficient for it; for we also need reasoning capacities, for example (those that allow us to unify our moral lives) in order to be morally unified.

According to the Unity View, the unity that a conscience promotes is a *moral* unity; what is at stake in choosing whether to act on our conscience is our *moral* integrity. Also, among our moral commitments, the ones that are most relevant to conscience are those that contribute to our moral identity (i.e., our "deep" moral commitments), because our psychological unity critically depends on whether we honor these commitments.[11] Failure to do so calls into question what kind of person we are, which can cause severe psychological rupture.

The moral unity that conscience encourages is also a unity not of predetermined or prescribed moral values, but rather of whatever moral values we happen to hold. In other words, the Unity View says that the deep moral commitments that inform our conscience are subjective rather than objective. Most bioethicists accept this fact (me included) and thus endorse what Kimberley Brownlee calls a "subjectivist" conception of conscience.[12] The reasons for doing so include skepticism that conscience could be "a little voice whispering to each of us infallibly about what we should do" (Sulmasy 2008, 136), together with the fact that understanding conscience objectively "would sound the death knell for conscientious objection in healthcare and the practice of accommodating health professionals with diverse [and often conflicting] conceptions of a morally decent life" (Wicclair 2017, 12). We would not consider providing such accommodation if we had an objectivist view about conscience.

Lastly, because the Unity View says that conscience functions to keep us in a certain relation to ourselves—one in which we have proper regard for and actively promote our moral integrity—the value it places on conscience is personal (Calhoun 1995, 252). Its value lies, more specifically, in us being personally integrated. And why does this unity have personal value? Advocates of the Unity View offer two basic answers. First, unity or inner peace contributes to our having a good life (Benjamin 2004, 470; Blustein 1993). Second, unity and the desire to repair "inner division" are admirable characteristics of persons (Blustein 1993, 297). This last response comes from Blustein. For him—and presumably for others—it is tempting to say of people who are internally divided that they owe it to themselves to try to become unified. That is true not simply because division can be difficult, but also because people would not be taking themselves seriously as moral

---

[11] One sees here the overlap between the Unity View and a view that connects conscience with an identity conception of integrity. See, again, note 1.

[12] Brownlee herself endorses a (secular) objectivist conception (2012).

agents if they thought little of acting against their moral principles or of having inconsistent principles. Here, Blustein suggests that we have a moral duty "to ourselves to lead personally integrated lives," and that in matters of inner unity, especially moral unity, our self-respect is at stake (1993, 297). On the Unity View then, moral integrity—understood as inner moral unity—is valuable because it promotes a good life as well as self-respect, and having a conscience is valuable because it encourages this unity.

1.2 Conscience and Inner Unity: How Strong Is the Connection?

On the whole, the Unity View says two things: 1) that acting with a conscience promotes inner unity, specifically moral unity; and 2) that the value of conscience just is the value of such unity. In what follows, I critically examine both of these claims.

Assuming that people can be unified to varying degrees, my discussion will focus on the degree of moral unity that a conscience is meant to foster on the Unity View: Is it perfect unity, optimal unity, or merely "serviceable" unity?[13] Advocates of the Unity View do not say.[14] But we need an answer if we are to understand how the Unity View connects conscience with inner unity. I consider all three levels of inner unity (perfect, optimal, and serviceable) and argue that conscience often does not function to support any of them, which means that its function and value must lie elsewhere. In defence of these points, I appeal to facts about people's social circumstances that are largely absent from the Unity View: in particular, to oppressive social relations that often influence what people value and in turn what makes them unified. These relations also shape people's ability to determine the meaning of what they have done and whether what they have done promotes or inhibits their inner unity. I propose that a careful consideration of such facts should lead us to question what the Unity View says about conscience and inner unity.

---

[13] The idea of a serviceable amount of unity comes from Margaret Walker. In discussing the concept of moral integrity, she writes that "more coherence, consistency, or continuity is not necessarily better...We need only so much as will serve" (Walker 1998, 115).

[14] Among advocates of the Unity View, Martin Benjamin is the only one who qualifies a statement about how much inner unity a conscience promotes; he states that having a conscience allows us to be "*reasonably* unified or integrated" (2004, 470; my emphasis). Unfortunately, he doesn't explain what he means by "reasonable." Is perfect unity reasonable? Is "reasonable" here a synonym for "optimal"?

Some clarity about the nature of inner unity is in order first. What does it actually mean to have inner unity, and more specifically, inner moral unity? According to Blustein, it means that our "actions and motivations [are in] harmony with our [moral] principles" (1993, 297; see also Benjamin 1995, 470). Presumably, our moral principles (and moral attitudes, etc.) would also have to be in harmony with one another, for otherwise we would be inconsistent or ambivalent, which are both marks of disunity. Inner unity, in addition, is something that we achieve through critical reflection or examination. As Benjamin says, "[t]he words, deeds, and convictions of an *unexamined* life are unlikely to be sufficiently integrated to constitute a singular life" (1995, 470; my emphasis).

Because moral principles, attitudes, and actions can be more or less in harmony with one another, inner unity must come in degrees. I have said that the Unity View is unclear about what degree of inner unity a conscience is meant to foster. Could it be perfect unity?

1.2.1 Perfect unity

Does our conscience aim to make us perfectly unified, so that we experience *no* ambivalence or inconsistency? Is a good conscience *completely* clean and easy? Would promoting perfect unity even make our conscience valuable?

I assume the answer to these questions is no, and imagine that advocates of the Unity View would agree with me. Perfect unity is a fantasy for beings like us, because not everything that we value or do is available to our consciousness so that we can unify it. Even if we were utterly transparent to ourselves, our moral lives would be too complex to admit of perfect unity. For to have perfect moral unity, there would need to be a clear ranking to our moral values, so that if they ever conflicted with one another (e.g., being honest conflicted with being compassionate), we would know exactly what to do to resolve the conflict. Most, if not all of us, lack such a moral system. Indeed, many of us frequently experience moral conflicts that admit of no clear solution (or no solution at all).[15] It follows that even if a state of perfect unity were possible for us, we would rarely be in it. Thus, it is reasonable to assume that the inner unity conscience promotes is not perfect. Consistently acting with a conscience will not allow us to achieve perfect unity, which is not to say, of course, that it will not enable us to be more unified than we would otherwise be.

---

[15] Marilyn Frye argues that is especially true of people who experience oppression (1983).

1.2.2 Optimal unity

If by "inner moral unity" advocates of the Unity View do not mean perfect unity, then perhaps they mean optimal unity. Moral unity is optimal if it is as much unity as we can hope for given the complexity of our moral lives. The Unity View would then amount to the claim that conscience promotes optimal moral unity and that the value of conscience just is the value of this unity, which itself promotes a good life and a good character.

Optimal inner unity can certainly be valuable. Aurora Levins Morales explains that it is valuable for political resistance, for example; she writes that resisters need to be "as whole as it is possible to be" for their resistance to be as powerful as it can be (Levins Morales 1998, 20). Speaking more generally, optimal unity can be important for psychological well-being, as well as for virtue.

It is still worth asking whether optimal inner unity is always valuable, and even whether our conscience normally encourages it. Surely such unity does not always contribute to a good life and a good character. To see why, consider a hypothetical nurse, Nurse B, a woman[16] who suffers from psychological oppression (Bartky 1990). Nurse B has low self-worth because she has internalized views about women being inferior and about nurses being nothing more than "intelligent machines" that exist "for the purpose of carrying out [doctor's] orders" (Benjamin and Curtis 1992, 22). Nurse B could be optimally unified around her low self-worth, in which case many of her actions and thoughts would be consistent with it. Her sense that as a woman, she matters relatively little, and that as a nurse, she contributes relatively little to patient care, would infect as much of her as possible, precisely *because* she is optimally unified around this diminished perception of herself. I assume that such unity is not good for her—it does not contribute to her having a good life—and that it is not something she (or anyone else) morally ought to encourage. Instead, she would have a better life and a better character if she were to oppose any internal pressure she feels (i.e., from her conscience) to be optimally unified in this way. It follows that optimal inner unity does not always promote a good life and a good character. It is not always valuable, and conscience would not always be valuable either if its value was tied to this degree of unity.

---

[16] I use terms like "woman" or "man" without specifying whether the people are cisgender or trans when I believe they could be either (which will make sense with some examples only if the trans women or men pass as being cisgender).

One might argue that the Unity View can explain the intuition that not all forms of optimal unity are worth protecting. For surely on this view, optimal inner unity or inner unity in general is not sufficient for a good life, which means that some unified lives may not be good.[17] Also, while moral integrity is a virtue, it is not the only virtue; it could be a bad thing on the Unity View that the inner unity of Nurse B comes at the expense of her self-respect, for example. For supporters of the Unity View to agree with these points, however, they would have to accept that optimal inner unity is valuable not always but other things being equal. In turn, they would have to believe that conscience is valuable other things being equal because the inner unity that it promotes may not be valuable. Yet I doubt that advocates of the Unity View could stomach this conclusion, since it implies that having a conscience can be worthless; according to them, stating that someone has a conscience *does* rather than *can* connote moral praise.

But let's leave these concerns aside and assume that the Unity View really is that conscience is valuable because it promotes optimal inner unity. The question remains: Does conscience actually have this effect? Next, I will give reasons for thinking that the answer is no. My focus there will be on whether the function and value of conscience lies in it preserving a serviceable amount of unity.

1.2.3 Serviceable unity

A serviceable moral unity is the minimal amount of unity that one needs to get on with life and be morally responsible. It is essential for moral agency, particularly for our ability to make moral choices, which we lose if we become wracked with guilt or shame and become unable to believe as a result that we are truly committed to anything. I assume that bringing about such extreme negative emotion is bad, even if it occurs while we are resisting oppression or the like. For instance, Nurse B could transgress norms about nurses being strictly obedient, but feel so horrible about it, so lost—as though her life no longer had meaning—that the transgression is not worth it.[18] It would be wrong of us to cheer her on in "misbehaving," as she would

---

[17] For example, we would hardly say of people who are optimally unified around an abusive and racist character that their lives are good, morally or otherwise. Thanks to an anonymous referee (of McLeod 2012) for alerting me to this objection.

[18] This scenario is consistent with the claim that some people will need to undergo radical change to free themselves of psychological oppression (Davion 1991). The scenario simply suggests that the change cannot happen so quickly, or in such a way, that it undermines our agency.

put it. Cases like hers suggest that serviceable moral unity is valuable and that having a conscience itself is valuable if it protects this degree of unity.

The idea that conscience functions to preserve serviceable unity coheres well with the Unity View, particularly with its emphasis on the dramatic language that can accompany an appeal to conscience, like "I wouldn't be able to live with myself" or "I couldn't look at myself in the mirror." Such phrases are well suited for people who wish to protect their moral agency and thus be unified to a serviceable degree. Perhaps the Unity View should be interpreted then as the view that conscience has value because it is needed for serviceable unity.

The question is whether the Unity View would then be correct. Does conscience function to preserve the minimal amount of unity that is needed for moral agency? There are at least two reasons for thinking that it does not.[19] Consider first that for conscience to play this role, our moral agency would actually have to be at stake when we do what our conscience says that we ought not to do. In other words, it would have to be *true* that we would not be able to live with ourselves if we ignored our conscience and committed acts that we thought were morally wrong. One might think that this claim is true of many of us, depending at least on what the relevant acts are: that if we killed another person, for example, we really would be unbearable to ourselves. Yet the empirical evidence indicates the opposite: that many of us could live with ourselves quite easily after committing acts we thought we would never commit. We are more resilient, in other words, than our dramatic claims ("I couldn't look at myself in the mirror") suggest. By putting the best spin on what we have done, or what we have learned because of what we have done, we can get along reasonably well most of the time (Gilbert 2006, Ch. 8).[20] Psychologist Daniel Gilbert argues that people are generally predisposed to think there is some goodness in what they have done when what they have done is bad (*very* bad even), because they want to believe

[19] Here's a third reason: our conscience can encourage us to honor commitments that are not deep enough to shake us to our moral core. I disagree with the Unity View that our conscience encourages us to adhere mainly to moral commitments that are deep. (Calhoun makes the same point when critiquing the identity conception of integrity; see note 1 and Calhoun 1995, 245.) To illustrate, my conscience could warn me that I will feel guilty if I tell a white lie, even though the relevant moral commitment ("Don't tell white lies") is shallow and I could live with myself comfortably if I violated it.

[20] As noted by an anonymous reviewer, this fact may not say anything interesting about what we ought to do. True. But it does say something about how unified we are, which is what matters according to the Unity View of conscience.

that their lives are going well.[21] To be sure, finding some goodness in what they have done can require that they downplay what *they* have done by denying responsibility for it (and saying, e.g., that they were only following orders or they were a different person when it happened). Childress writes that someone who makes an appeal to conscience "claims that he will not be able to deny that the act is his if he performs it" (1979, 324). Indeed, that may be what this person claims, yet he could very well do the opposite if his only available route to mental well-being is to take little responsibility for the act in question.

People are limited, of course, in how much positive spin they can put on their actions or the actions of others. ("When our team's defensive tackle is caught wearing brass knuckles…we find it difficult to overlook or forget such facts"; Gilbert 2006, 168.) How limited people are in this regard, more-over, can depend on their social position (among other factors, of course). People who are privileged, for instance, tend to have more power than others to make their behavior seem benign or good, which is a point Paul Benson makes about men in sexist societies: "Men who reap advantages from [sexist social] arrangements are commonly in a position to justify their conduct by appealing to gendered social norms that grant men special prerogatives ('Lighten up! Surely there is nothing wrong in my just looking, teasing…') or by professing their innocent motives ('I didn't mean any harm by it')" (2000, 72). By contrast, women often lack the power to say, "lighten up," or to convince others, in certain contexts at least, that they "didn't mean any harm by [what they have done]." For instance, people tend not to believe a woman when she says she meant no harm in poking fun at someone who was deeply offended by her remarks. Such disbelief stems from the thought that as a woman—someone who is meant to be in tune with others' feelings—she could not have failed to understand the effect her words would have. She must have willed it to happen; she must have meant to cause the offence.

In short, people who are socially powerful can often convince others of their innocence or deflect blame onto others when they fail to do what their conscience dictates. With such authority, they can live with themselves quite peacefully despite ignoring their conscience. Although they might say they are loath to rely on this power, they might use it regardless, because they are psychologically disposed to try to be happy (or simply to maintain their

---

[21] No one who is psychologically healthy wants their life to go badly or to believe that's the case, which is at least partly why people tend to adapt quickly to negative changes in their environment (Gilbert 2006, 162).

power). It follows that their serviceable inner unity is not obviously at stake when they decide whether to listen to their conscience, and therefore, their conscience may not function at all to preserve their serviceable inner unity.

Perhaps *repeated* violations of conscience would put the serviceable inner unity of people in power at risk? This question is germane to discussions about conscience protection for health care professionals, who will likely receive repeated requests for any service to which they conscientiously object.[22] Imagine objecting physicians who refer all patients who want abortions to abortion providers; their conscience opposes this action, but their profession requires it. They might be able to spin making a referral positively the first time they do it, but will they be able to do so for each successive referral? Will the referrals not wear on them over time, and leave them full of regret? I suspect that they could do so, although the physicians could also receive enough social support in thinking that they are not complicit in an immoral act that they could keep their conscience relatively quiet. If no one else seriously questions how they define their behavior, which might happen because of their privilege, then they could certainly fail to question it themselves.

We have seen that people who have the power to cast themselves and their actions in positive light may be able to live with themselves despite *not listening* to their conscience. Consider now that the opposite is also true: that people who lack social power may not be able to live with themselves despite *listening* to their conscience. In other words, they put their serviceable inner unity at risk by heeding the dictates of their conscience, rather than by ignoring them. In that case, instead of protecting their inner unity, their conscience disrupts it. This point provides a second reason for thinking that conscience may not function to preserve our serviceable unity.

Here is an example, inspired by Lois Jensen, who launched the first sexual harassment case in the United States.[23] A woman charges her male co-workers with sexual harassment in an intensely sexist work environment, hoping that someone in power will take her complaint seriously, but nobody does. Having learned of her complaint, her male co-workers harass her even more, insisting that she is just an angry b----. Her female co-workers are too afraid to back her up, thinking that if they do, they will lose their jobs

---

[22] Thanks to Sara Goering for raising this important objection (in personal conversation).

[23] The legal case is *Jenson v Eveleth Taconite Co.*, 139 FRD 657 (D Minn 1991). The film *North Country* is based on Jenson's story (Caro 2005). Jenson won her legal battle and so was redeemed in the end. But, of course, there are cases like hers of sexual harassment that do not turn out so well, and in which women's lives are ruined because of how other people reacted to their complaints. My fictional scenario resembles cases like these.

and the harassment they face will increase. The woman is left with few supporters, with constant harassment, and with serious threats to her physical security. Imagine as well that she cannot quit her job because it is the only job she can get that allows her to care financially for her children. This woman listened to her conscience, but may be less morally unified and even lose serviceable unity as a result. She may not be able to persist in believing that by her own lights, what she has done is morally right. Instead, she might think that all she has done is made herself into a pariah in her community: someone who now must fear for her safety and that of her children. Alternatively, others' negative stories about her behavior may come to seem reasonable to her (she really is an angry b----). It would be hard if not impossible for her to sustain her own story if everyone else's was different. In that case, she would end up full of self-loathing and regret, with less moral unity than she started out with or no serviceable unity at all.

This example reveals the extent to which social support and the power to determine the meaning of what one has done (e.g., been disloyal as opposed to courageous) can shape people's experience of a conscientious refusal. The experience may be one of brokenness rather than unity, even serviceable unity. The Unity View cannot account for this fact without appreciating that people are embedded in social relations that influence how successful their attempts at moral action can be. The relevant social relations need not even be oppressive, since people who are not oppressed can listen to their conscience but then seriously regret it, because of how much it costs them socially (McLeod and Fitzgerald 2015, 349). This theme is common among whistleblowers, for example, regardless of their (initial) social position;[24] and it may arise for conscientious objectors in health care whose moral views are deeply unpopular.

One might object that it is implicit within the Unity View that without some social support for one's conscience, acting with a conscience can undermine one's inner unity. Advocates of this view argue in favor of social support for the conscience of health care professionals so that the professionals will not have to choose between stiff inner (i.e., personal) sanctions if they act without a conscience and stiff outer (i.e., social) sanctions if they act with a conscience. The hidden message is that acting with a conscience

---

[24] C. Fred Alford explains that many whistleblowers wish they had never taken the stand they did, because it cost them too much and had no effect on the organization they worked for (2001, 34). Many of his examples involve people who were not socially marginalized until they became whistleblowers. (For a discussion of "[w]hat happens when whistleblowers are also members of an oppressed group," see DesAutels 2009.)

can be devastating if the outer sanctions are too great. To respond, this insight might be shared among defenders of the Unity View, but notice it is inconsistent with the claim that our conscience functions (on its own anyway) to support our serviceable unity. It is not obviously compatible with the Unity View, so understood.

To conclude, I have cast doubt on whether conscience promotes serviceable unity or any other degree of inner unity for that matter. If it does not serve this function in a whole range of cases, then its function must lie elsewhere. Unlike with perfect and optimal unity, I have not questioned whether serviceable unity is always valuable. Instead, I have suggested that for some people—particularly those with social power—acting against their conscience often will not put their serviceable unity at serious risk, which means that doing the opposite—acting with a conscience—could not be required for their inner unity. For other people—those with little social power (or power within an organization)—acting *with* a conscience can undermine their serviceable unity, or at least disturb rather than promote their inner unity in general. On the whole, the connection the Unity View draws between such conduct and the preservation of one's integrity is therefore highly tenuous.

2. The Dynamic View

Despite the criticisms I've made, one might think the Unity View still has much to recommend it. After all, people who act on their conscience and feel justified in doing so will be optimally unified, at least at the time of acting. Having listened to their conscience, the majority of them could also be more unified long term than they otherwise would be. That may include some people who face severe social sanctions because of their conscientious action; objectors who are sanctioned with inhumane treatment can still feel as though they did the right thing.

I agree that there may be some truth to the Unity View; nonetheless, I doubt that it is the correct view. I will contend that conscience functions not to preserve inner unity, but to encourage us simply to act on our moral values. What is more, the value of conscience goes beyond its function, rather than being identical to it, which is what the Unity View suggests. Conscience has value potentially when it urges us to take our moral values seriously, but also when it forces us to reconsider and revise some of those values, after perhaps clarifying for us what they are. Our conscience can alert us to how deeply committed we are to certain values, and can prompt us, in turn, to embrace different values. Notice that here, the function and value of conscience must come apart; it would be inconsistent to say that conscience functions to get us to reconsider doing what it simultaneously encourages us to do (i.e., act on values that we hold deeply). Still, the value of conscience could lie in this after-effect of conscience (i.e., in the urge to rethink some of what we value). Let me expand on these points, which inform my Dynamic View of conscience. Then I'll use this theory to explain what is at stake in denying conscience protection to health care professionals.

My understanding of the function of conscience—that it encourages us to do what we think we morally ought to do—is relatively uncontroversial. It fits with ideas about conscience that appear in most if not all theories of conscience, including the Unity View. The motivating idea is that conscience "influences (but rarely, if ever completely controls) [one's] conduct" and that at bottom, conscience is "a capacity...to sense or immediately discern that what [one] has done, is doing, or is about to do (or not do) is wrong, bad, and worthy of disapproval" (Hill 1998, 14). This second idea tells us that the voice of conscience is often negative; it arises when we believe we deserve blame rather than praise. In this sense, it encourages us to do what we think we morally ought to do by actively discouraging us from doing the opposite.

Elizabeth Kiss calls our conscience our "inner nag" (1998, 69). Our conscience nags us into doing what we think we morally ought to do but are somewhat averse to doing. Although a conscience and a nag may be dissimilar in some respects,[25] the two have much in common. For example, a nag continually harasses us when we wish just to be left alone; and similarly, our conscience pesters us when we try to ignore it and do what we please.[26] The voice comes unbidden, especially when we persist in doing or planning to do what we feel is morally wrong (Hill 1998). In this way, our conscience differs from our conscious moral judgment; we have more control over whether we make such judgments than we do over whether our conscience affects us (which, in turn, limits how dynamic our conscience can be). As on the Unity View, on the Dynamic View, conscience and moral judgment are not identical. The Dynamic View is unique, however, in insisting that conscience and moral judgment can and should influence one another.

---

[25] For example, a nag is often ineffective, while a conscience can be very effective, that is, in getting us to do what we think we morally ought to do. I owe this point to Jennifer Nedelsky (personal communication).

[26] Unlike on the Unity View, on my view, conscience rarely threatens us with complete psychic dissolution. A nag is not as menacing as that. Our conscience lacks this quality in general because often it encourages us to adhere to moral commitments that are not deep. See note 18.

I have said that the function of conscience is simply to encourage us to take our moral values seriously. But if conscience works this way, then many of us will be skeptical of its value. The reason why is that for many people, their "inner nag" is sexist, racist, or oppressive in other ways. Because of our enmeshment within oppressive social structures, many of us are internally compelled to act in ways that are oppressive to others or to ourselves. For example, some LGBTQ+ people feel internal pressure to participate in their own oppression by conforming to prevailing gender norms (see, e.g., Calhoun 1995), revealing that at some level, they are committed to these norms. I assume that if we hold a subjectivist view of conscience, then we must accept that people's ability to discern that they are not acting in accordance with moral commitments of this kind (or of any kind) is conscience. But then we must ask, why really should we value this capacity?

I think there are two reasons, in fact, why we should value conscience. First, the voice of it will not always be one of internalized oppression, for sometimes our conscience will reflect what we genuinely believe to be correct. Second, even when our conscience is a voice of oppression (or abuse or the like), it can have a positive effect, that is, by alerting us to having some oppressive or otherwise bad values that may be unconsciously influencing our behavior. To illustrate, my conscience could encourage me to prepare dinner for my husband most nights, simply because he is my husband. It would do that by threatening me with false guilt or shame (Taylor 1987), which are emotions that do not reflect what I actively endorse. The relevant values would, in that sense, be alien to me; although they would not be entirely alien, since they obviously find some expression in me. My conscience would allow me to see how much these values are a part of me and could prompt me to reflect on how I was relating to my spouse because of them. Say that I'd been making his dinner repeatedly, but then wanted a break from it. Taking a break is not as easy as I thought it would be, because my conscience starts to nag me about preparing dinner. I say to myself, "But why should I feel guilty about not making dinner? Do I really believe that I ought to be making his dinner, because I'm his wife? Maybe deep down, I do accept that, which is troubling to say the least. I should reject these attitudes and resist getting into patterns of "wifely" behavior, rather than allow them to develop." Notice the positive role that conscience plays in this story. By making me aware of values that influence my behavior—negatively in my opinion—it helps me to take responsibility for myself (Card 1996), and for how I am structuring my intimate relationships with others. This example shows how conscience can aid us in retooling ourselves morally and in developing more authentic moral selves, ones that are informed by our moral judgments.[27]

Retooling ourselves morally involves remaking our conscience so that it threatens us with *genuine* guilt or shame, rather than the false variety. This happy outcome would occur when judgments about what we morally ought to value sink in, changing what we do value, and thereby altering what our conscience warns us about (a process that has important social elements to it, as I discuss further on in this section). A conscience like this is *dynamic* in the following sense: it will change when it conflicts with what we judge to be morally correct. On this view, our moral judgment can influence our conscience, but our conscience can also influence our moral judgment. It does so when it jump-starts the process of moral retooling.

While the Dynamic View emphasizes the importance of people reflecting on the judgments that inform their conscience, the Unity View says relatively little in this regard. Granted, the Unity View is not as extreme as some religious views that instruct us to live our lives in conformity with our conscience without questioning what it says. Advocates of the Unity View do accept that at times we should scrutinize the demands of our conscience.[28] But they do not associate the value of conscience with its ability to inspire attempts at taking responsibility for what we value.

The process of retooling our conscience so that it comes closer to what we reflectively endorse has important social dimensions to it. We need social relations that give us a vision of the world that is a positive alternative to the one we have internalized: that can create or confirm a suspicion in us that what we have learned is false. For instance, I learned that as a cisgendered woman, I ought to nurture men and children in the ways of a fairly traditional wife and mother. Although I rebelled to some extent, I did not feel confident in my rebellion until I went to university and started taking courses in feminist philosophy. This experience did not rid me of oppressive influences—when I met my spouse, I still wanted to nurture him as my mother did my father—still, it marked the beginning of my "moral makeover," so to speak. The makeover continues with help from my spouse, who,

---

[27] I owe the phrase "retool ourselves morally" to Sheila Wildeman (personal communication). By the term "authentic," I simply mean in accordance with our best judgment, which itself is never free from social influence.

[28] Childress says we need to do so when we experience a "crisis of conscience," that is, when our conscience gives us multiple demands that conflict (1979, 320). Blustein says that we could, although need not necessarily, do so after having violated a demand of our conscience; we might reconsider the adequacy of the demand in light of what motivated us to ignore it ("sympathies, longings, fears, anxieties, etc."; 1993, 296).

like me, resists the "gendering of our relationship" (his phrase). This example illustrates how our relations with others, especially intimate ones, can shape not only who we are, but also who we try to become. Most of us cannot retool ourselves, or aspects of ourselves such as our conscience, all by ourselves.

To recapitulate, according to the Dynamic View, conscience has value when it encourages us not simply to do what we think we morally ought to do, but also to revise those thoughts when necessary to give voice to what we genuinely value. On this view, a conscience is dynamic when it reflects our moral endorsements, while at the same time influencing what those endorsements are. Although a conscience could instead be "the echo of social and parental admonitions" (Benjamin 1995, 470), it needn't be that, or only that.

The question remains, why does conscience have value insofar as it prompts us to do what we truly believe to be morally right? My answer is reminiscent of the Unity View: having a conscience of this sort promotes our moral integrity. "Integrity" here is understood, not as inner unity, however, but as abiding by one's best judgment (in this case, moral judgment). This conception of integrity, which I have defended elsewhere (McLeod 2004; 2005), comes from Cheshire Calhoun (1995), who insists that integrity is importantly different from inner unity. According to Calhoun, honoring our best judgment will not necessarily promote our inner unity, because our best judgment about our situation may be that different values are at stake and that they cannot be reconciled. In addition, the process of coming to decide what our best judgment is may cause us to question much of what we had previously taken for granted, which will destabilize us, at least initially, more than it will unify us. Taking responsibility for our moral selves, which is what moral integrity requires, is not the same as striving for moral consistency.[29]

The above account of integrity is similar to, yet distinct from, one that Mark Wicclair defends (2000; 2011; 2017). For Wicclair, integrity centers on *identity* rather than inner unity (2017).[30] In his view, having integrity involves acting on beliefs that are "integral" to our self-understanding and that we "are disposed to explicitly endorse," regardless, presumably, of

---

[29] Recall that Blustein argues that inner unity is valuable because it reveals a desire on the part of moral agents to take themselves seriously as moral agents. One lacks this desire if one thinks little of acting against one's moral principles or of having inconsistent principles. But I question whether having inner unity is the same as having the above desire. One could achieve inner unity (of an optimal sort) by adhering to whatever moral commitments one happens to hold so long as they are consistent. People who take themselves seriously as moral agents, however, would be critical of moral commitments they just happen to hold.

[30] See notes 1 and 6.

whether we achieve greater inner unity as a result (2011, 5). Since acting on beliefs of this sort could amount to acting on our best moral judgment, Wicclair's theory is similar to Calhoun's. Still, there are at least three important differences between the two. First, integrity focuses on identity for Wicclair but not for Calhoun, who claims that acting on one's best judgment can involve acting on beliefs that are not identity-conferring (Calhoun 1995, 245; see also note 18). Second, the moral beliefs that concern our integrity are quite static for Wicclair, but not for Calhoun. Wicclair insists that our identity-conferring moral beliefs "tend to be persistent and subject to change only in response to significant life events, such as near death experiences, tragic events, and extreme changes in fortune," and they also "tend to be resistant to influence by others" (5). By contrast, Calhoun is open to our moral judgments being quite dynamic and responsive to others' influence—particularly to attempts by others to help us to decide on what our best judgment is. In this way, her theory coheres well with the Dynamic View of conscience. Finally, Calhoun argues that adhering to our best judgment in a way that promotes our integrity has social value rather than merely personal value, while Wicclair rejects the idea that integrity has this "social component" (2017, 9–11). Whether integrity indeed has social value is not an issue I can settle here; nonetheless, let me briefly describe why I find this view compelling.

There is personal value to living an authentic moral life—value that is linked with self-respect and a lack of self-betrayal—but there is also social value in people taking their own best moral judgment seriously. Society needs this commitment from people so that genuine debates about moral right and wrong can occur, which themselves are important because they help to improve our moral understanding (Calhoun 1995; Mill 1851/1989; McLeod 2005, 126). On this view, gaining moral knowledge is a social process (Calhoun 1995; Walker 1998) and integrity has social value, because it contributes to this process.[31] Insofar as conscience encourages people to act with integrity, so understood, it also can have social value. It has this value when it encourages people to feel genuine guilt or shame, that is, upon

---

[31] This point reveals that the production of moral knowledge depends on integrity, but is the reverse also true? In other words, does having integrity involve participating in the social process of knowledge production? The answer is yes, because integrity involves "standing for something," which one does only "for, and before,...deliberators who share the goal of determining what is worth doing" (Calhoun 1995, 257). Wicclair misses this point in a critique he offers of Calhoun's theory (2017, 10). He suggests that she fails to show a "*conceptual* connection" between integrity and participating in an evaluative community. Yet I believe the connection appears clearly in the final section of her paper (section V) and in her title, "Standing for Something" (1995).

failing to respect their best moral judgment. This explanation informs my Dynamic View of conscience, according to which the value of conscience can be social as well as personal.

Clearly, on my view, not everyone's conscience will have the same value (i.e., social and personal value). People who abide by their conscience, even when its message is inconsistent with what they do or would endorse (e.g., if they were free of psychological oppression), will have a conscience with little value to it. People who do *not* defer to the conscience they simply find themselves with and who change some of their moral commitments, but do so without having good reasons for making those changes, will also have a conscience with little value to it. Among the latter, I count people who retool themselves so that their moral values become more oppressive than they were before, which is possible given the noxious social environments that people can become immersed in later in life. I assume that when asked to explain these types of changes, people "invariably come up short" (McLeod 2004, 228; Piper 1990; Appiah 1990). It may be that their conscience is still worth something, for simply having a conscience means that they care about doing what is morally right, as they perceive it, which is better than not caring at all. Still, their conscience must be worth substantially less than it would be if they had values they could support. The moral judgments that influence their conscience would add little to social debate about the nature of right and wrong.

Hopefully by now it is clear that the Dynamic View of conscience is preferable to the Unity View in terms of how it describes the value of conscience. It makes sense of intuitions about its value that many of us share, but that the Unity View cannot explain: that the conscience of the subjugated nurse from Section 1 has little value (for the values that inform her conscience are oppressive to her), that the conscience of someone who is completely unreflective morally also has little value, and that acting with a conscience can have value even when it does not unify us (for the value might be purely social, which could be the case with the woman from Section 1 who resists workplace harassment).[32] The conception of conscience that informs discussion about conscience in bioethics should, I believe, cohere with these intuitions.

---

[32] It might not be the case for this woman, however. She might come to value what she did after becoming immersed in a social context that acknowledges sexual harassment to be a crime.

The Dynamic View has a lot to tell us about when and how we ought to value conscience in health care. Let me wrap up this chapter by summarizing this advice.

2.1 When to Value Conscience

In answer to when (if ever) we should be concerned about protecting the conscience of objecting health care professionals, advocates of the Unity View would say "always." Their explanation would be that the inner unity—and ultimately the self-respect and personal welfare—of these professionals is at stake. As we have seen, however, this answer is problematic when the relevant unity centers on values that are oppressive (recall Nurse B). We should *not* be concerned with protecting conscience in these cases, and the Dynamic View explains why that is true. It says that when conscience is a stagnant reminder of internalized oppression, rather than a reflection of our best moral judgment, it is worth very little, if anything at all.[33] We should be concerned about the conscience of health care professionals, according to this view, when these professionals have the sort of dynamic conscience I've described. In that case, there are important values at stake in denying them the ability to act on their conscience: namely, the personal value of them leading an authentic moral life and the social value of them contributing to social debate about what's worth doing in health care.

Moving forward, we could assume that most conscientious objectors in health care lack a conscience of any value, but that would be uncharitable. I'll assume instead that many, if not most objectors, have a dynamic conscience: one that is responsive to their reflective moral judgment or responsive enough that we should take their appeals to conscience seriously. I include within this group many of the typical conscientious objectors in reproductive health care, who again refuse to provide standard services like abortions out of concern for the lives of the fetuses or embryos. Although these

---

[33] Whether the conscience of health care professionals reflect their best moral judgment should be evident from their responses to questions about why they have the conscience they do, or why they need to conscientiously refuse to provide a certain service. Professionals whose conscience is informed by their autonomous judgment should be able to give a decent answer to this question (i.e., an answer other than "I simply believe that's the case"). This point speaks in favor of having conscientious objectors in health care explain their objections to employers or licensing boards, rather than allowing them to object without explanation (see Kantymir and McLeod 2014; Marsh 2014; Card 2007; Downie 2012). Although I don't advocate for such a position, my view about the value of conscience does support it.

refusals can reinforce sexism or other forms of oppression as I explain in Chapter 2, they are not obviously prompted by oppressive values. Instead, what may, and I assume does, often motivate them is the objector's best moral judgment about when "human life begins" and about how valuable such lives are relative to patients' interests in obtaining the reproductive services they seek.

2.2 How to Value Conscience

There are lessons to be drawn from this chapter about how (vs. when) to value conscience in health care. For example, because acting with a conscience can have both social and personal value, the culture of health care institutions should not be hostile toward individual conscience. There should be some openness, in particular, to the conscience of professionals who have minority views, who are members of marginalized social groups, or who are powerless relative to physicians or administrators.[34] At the same time, valuing the conscience of health care professionals does not require that we permit conscientious refusals. For example, we can promote the social value of their conscience by ensuring that they can freely express their moral opposition to the status quo at venues where policy decisions get made, rather than in their interactions with patients.

In addition, because of the dynamic side of conscience on the Dynamic View, we should not assume that the conscience of health care professionals is fixed and thus not amenable to change through health ethics education.[35] Respecting the conscience of health care professionals is perfectly compatible, on this view, with trying to convince them of the moral wisdom behind what is the standard of care.

3. Conclusion

This chapter has focused on the value of conscience, which is relevant to whether conscientious refusals in health care actually pose a serious moral

---

[34] Of course, there ought to be protection also for the conscience of patients, as I suggest in this book, particularly in Chapters 2 and 5.

[35] The point that we should avoid such an assumption comes from Carolyn Ells (personal communication).

problem. I have claimed that conscience (or acting with a conscience) can indeed have value, and in going forward, I will assume this value is manifest in many cases of conscientious refusal, including typical cases in reproductive health care. I have argued that the value of conscience is best illuminated by the Dynamic View rather than Unity View. According to the former, its value comes in degrees and is highest when our conscience is dynamic and most reflects our best moral judgment, and lowest when our conscience just parrots moral principles we have absorbed in our society. Whether we have a conscience of high or low value will depend somewhat on our social relations, which can affect how motivated we are to retool our conscience so that the guilt or shame it threatens us with is genuine. A conscience that is dynamic in this way is an important source of moral integrity, which itself has social and personal value.

If I am correct that conscience can have substantial value and often has such value among health care professionals, then we should not take lightly the prospect of restricting their freedom of conscience. I argue for serious restrictions of this sort in this book, but only when conscience conflicts with what is standard of care. I do so with full acknowledgment of the value conscience can have in health care and with the insistence that unless their conscience is valueless (e.g., it is racist or sexist), we should not, without good reason, deny health care professionals the ability to act on their conscience.

2

Harm or Mere Inconvenience?

As revealed in Chapter 1, conscientious refusals in health care are a serious moral issue. One U.S. commentator even names the issue the "San Andreas Fault of [U.S.] culture...How we decide this is going to have a long-lasting impact on our society" (Stein 2006). The impact, good or bad, will be most severe on parties who are directly involved in conflicts of conscience in health care: namely, patients who are denied standard services, and professionals who conscientiously object to providing them. Chapter 1 dealt with what's at stake with these conflicts for the professionals who object, while the current chapter, along with Chapter 3, examine what's at stake for the patients who are denied treatment, particularly in reproductive health care contexts. The goal of these chapters is to show that something important is indeed at stake for many, if not most, of these patients. This fact explains why policymakers should consider carefully whether to allow conscientious refusals in reproductive health care.

What is the likely impact on patients of being denied health care services by a conscientiously objecting professional? They obviously will not get the services they seek right away. Yet as commentators often point out—in discussions about conscientious objection in *reproductive* health care in particular—the patients could simply go to another clinic or hospital to get this care, especially if they live in an area where the relevant services are available somewhere else. The conclusion we are invited to accept is that these patients are merely inconvenienced rather than harmed when they encounter a conscientiously objecting professional, which if true would mean that the impact on the patient in many cases of conscientious refusal is not morally significant. I argue in this chapter that this claim about inconvenience is seriously mistaken.

This book concentrates mainly on services in reproductive health care that objectors refuse to provide on the grounds that the services end, or put in jeopardy, the lives of embryos or fetuses. Such refusals are typical ones. Although the argument I make in this chapter extends to all typical refusals, it focuses on refusals that pharmacists make to providing emergency

Conscience in Reproductive Health Care: Prioritizing Patient Interests. Carolyn McLeod, Oxford University Press (2020).
© Carolyn McLeod.
DOI: 10.1093/oso/9780198732723.001.0001

contraception (EC) (pharmacists being the usual gatekeepers of EC).[1] I narrow the discussion in this way because the best defense in the literature of the claim that patients are merely inconvenienced by conscientious refusals in reproductive health care comes from authors who center their attention on pharmacist refusals to offer EC. The authors I have in mind are Elizabeth Fenton and Loren Lomasky (2005) (hereafter "F&L"). Contra F&L, I say that it is more plausible to conclude that being denied EC on grounds of conscience harms many patients rather than inconveniencing them,[2] and that is true even if the patients could get EC somewhere else nearby. As I briefly demonstrate, the same argument applies to patients who are denied an abortion by a conscientious objector who is a gatekeeper of this service.

To be clear, my objective in this chapter is not to try to resolve conflicts of conscience in reproductive health care; their dimensions, like those of the San Andreas Fault, are too vast to cope with in a short space. Instead, I simply deal with one side of them: that of the patient requesting care, especially basic reproductive health care. What I say about this side does factor into an argument I give later about how these conflicts should be settled (see esp. Chapter 5). More specifically, my claim here—that typical refusals in reproductive health care cause harm rather than mere inconvenience to many patients—helps to support the prioritizing approach I take later to these refusals.

1. A Mere Inconvenience

Let me turn to the typical refusals that are the focus on this chapter: refusals by pharmacists to dispense EC. Pro-life people who support pharmacists in such action tend to see patients' ability to obtain EC as a matter of mere convenience, which in turn allows them to deny the severity of conflicts of conscience in pharmaceutical practice. "Should one person's convenience

---

[1] That is particularly true of the EC levonorgestrel (Plan B), which is now available without a prescription, and therefore directly from pharmacists, in over eighty countries (Schulz et al. 2016). In most of these countries, the drug remains behind the counter, and thus patients must request it from a pharmacist.

[2] Another possibility is that they are wronged but are neither harmed nor inconvenienced. The assumption here is that there are wrongs that are not harms. (Later on, I discuss the opposite: harms that are not wrongs.) People are wronged but not harmed, at least "*on balance,*" if they mostly benefit from a wrong (e.g., their land is improved by having someone trespass on it; Feinberg 1984, 35; his emphasis). Since it would be rare that on balance, a patient would benefit from being denied EC, I will not consider any further the possibility that in general, patients are wronged but not harmed by this experience.

trump another person's moral conscience? That's obnoxious, offensive and un-American," says one pro-life commentator (Laugminas 2005; cited in Vischer 2006, 93). The view here could be that acquiring EC is a mere convenience, because EC is not a medically necessary service; in other words, patients do not need it but rather prefer it, and so are only inconvenienced if they cannot get it. Alternatively, the view could be that accessing EC is a mere convenience only when the request for it is directed toward a particular pharmacist—one who will not or cannot provide it—and there are other pharmacists nearby who would dispense it. In other words, it is a mere convenience to obtain it from the first pharmacist one approaches. Of these positions, pro-life people tend to take the former, but I'm interested in the latter, which exists in the literature on conscientious refusals among theorists who have no moral objection to EC. I have in mind in particular F&L (2005), but also Robert K. Vischer (2006).[3]

To be fair to F&L, they support some restrictions on the right of pharmacists to conscientiously refuse to provide EC, though not because they feel that these refusals harm patients (or "clients" as they call them).[4] The view that they defend is actually quite complex. To help explain it, I've devised some conditionals that F&L themselves do not construct but that they would accept and that concern whether pharmacists' conscientious refusals are indeed harmful. Here are the conditionals:[5]

1)   If patients who requested EC faced a true emergency, then being refused it by a pharmacist would harm them.

2)   If patients who sought EC were entitled to get it from any pharmacist, because every pharmacist had a duty to dispense EC to any patient who makes a legitimate request for it, then being refused EC by a pharmacist would harm them.

---

[3] Vischer writes that having to "drive across town" to obtain EC is a "market-driven inconvenience" (113). Another author who makes a similar claim is Holly Fernandez Lynch (2008), although she does not focus her attention on EC.

[4] I employ the term "patient" because it has become widely accepted within pharmacy (Austin et al. 2006). There is controversy surrounding its use in this context, to be sure, but the same is true about the term "client."

[5] I've left out one conditional: if patients who were denied EC were browbeaten or otherwise harassed by the pharmacist, then they would be harmed. F&L would agree with this conditional as well (F&L 2005, 584). In addition, they appear to believe that at most *some* patients are browbeaten or harassed, and are harmed for this reason by conscientious refusals. I leave cases of this sort aside and focus on ones where there is a simple conscientious refusal, with no harassment or even attempts at moral persuasion. My reasons are twofold: (1) we simply do not know how common harassment and moral persuasion are in this context; and (2) it is worthwhile demonstrating that even simple refusals tend to cause harm.

3) If patients who asked for EC were entitled to get it from some pharmacists, because some (not all) pharmacists have a duty to dispense it, then being refused EC by one of these pharmacists would harm them.

With respect to 1) and 2), F&L deny that patients requesting EC confront a true emergency and that every pharmacist has a duty to dispense it. They also assume that only if these claims are true could every patient who is refused EC by a pharmacist be harmed by this experience. At the same time, they accept that some of these patients could be harmed, since F&L believe—and this is relevant to 3)—that some pharmacists have a duty to dispense EC. My goal will be to show that in arguing for these points, F&L employ an overly narrow conception of harm, but that even if this conception was correct, their reasoning against the view that conscientious refusals are always harmful would be flawed.

First let me describe in some detail how F&L would respond to each conditional.

1) If patients who requested EC faced a true emergency, then being refused it by a pharmacist would harm them.

F&L would agree with this statement on the following grounds. Like other professionals, pharmacists are obligated to provide services in emergency situations (F&L 2005, 582). They would therefore be required to dispense EC, and patients would be entitled to receive it from them, *if* needing EC constituted a true emergency. When people do not get that to which they are entitled, they are harmed. Denying patients EC would therefore harm them.

Importantly, F&L do not accept that patients requesting EC face a true emergency or that it is legitimate for us to assume that they do. They write: "[S]o long as other sources are willing to step in, the case falls under the category of convenience rather than emergency" (582). They go on to say that classifying the case of patients seeking EC as an emergency even when there are no other sources willing to step in is illegitimate. For, "whether averting an unwanted pregnancy can ever count as an emergency is precisely the crux of the parties' dispute. The pharmacist who insists on a right of conscientious refusal maintains that it is the nascent human life that is in dire jeopardy, not the prospective mother" (F&L 2005, 582). Thus, unless we are to decide the case in favor of the patient at the outset, we should avoid calling the patient's situation an emergency. F&L argue further, with respect to refusals to dispense EC, that the patients may not get pregnant anyway, or if they do, could have an abortion, and so there is no emergency in terms of them being forced to become a "mother" (582).

2) If patients who sought EC were entitled to get it from any pharmacist, because every pharmacist had a duty to dispense EC to any patient who makes a legitimate request for it, then being refused EC by a pharmacist would harm them.

F&L would agree to this conditional on the grounds that denying people that to which they are entitled harms them.

Yet F&L do not believe that every pharmacist has a duty to dispense EC to every patient who makes a legitimate request for it (i.e., a request made for legitimate medical reasons). They give two reasons for this: a) like physicians and other professionals, pharmacists enjoy the freedom to "choose whom to serve,"[6] at least in non-emergency situations; and this freedom is inconsistent with a duty to dispense (F&L 2005, 582). b) As individual citizens, pharmacists have no duty to aid others, only a duty of noninterference (584).[7] This second, libertarian premise helps to bolster F&L's claim that patients seeking EC are not entitled to get it from individual pharmacists on the grounds that there is a "duty to treat" in pharmacy (see, e.g., Arras 1988; Clark 2005); on their view, there could be no harm to these patients that exists because of their being denied services to which they are entitled, again on these grounds.

F&L say that rather than being harmed, a patient who requests EC but is turned away is merely denied a benefit. In their words:

> She is inconvenienced in pursuing her ends and may experience discomfort
> at being branded a moral transgressor, this at a time when she is especially

---

[6] This language comes from the *Principles of Medical Ethics* of the American Medical Association (2016). Principle VI of this document reads: "A physician shall, in the provision of appropriate patient care, except in emergencies, be free to choose whom to serve, with whom to associate, and the environment in which to provide medical service." F&L assume that pharmacists have the same right. I return to it later in this chapter and also in Chapter 6.

[7] It is unclear whether this second claim is a moral or a legal one. F&L acknowledge arguments to the effect that everyone has a duty to be a Minimally Decent Samaritan (Thomson 1971) and that those who are "specially qualified" to provide the necessary aid (e.g., health professionals) may be required to be more than just minimally decent (Clark 2005, 79; see F&L 2005, note 5, 590–1). But F&L dismiss these arguments on the grounds that they refer to moral duties, rather than legal or professional duties, as though F&L were not concerned with moral duties. In other parts of their paper, however, they seem obviously concerned with morality, including parts where they discuss a duty to aid; for example, they say that a "failure to render aid is [not] *morally* on all fours with the infliction of harm" (583, my emphasis).

vulnerable. Moreover, that vulnerability can be transformed, by refusal, into an unwanted pregnancy. But...these considerations nonetheless fall short of demonstrating the occurrence of an actionable harm. By refusing to enter into a transaction that the other party desires, one thereby *fails to provide a benefit* but [does] not...*inflict a liability* [i.e., a harm].

(F&L 2005, 583; their emphasis)

To continue with F&L's reasoning: one would inflict harm only if one was obliged to deal with the other party in a certain manner and yet refused to do so. But individual pharmacists are not obliged to accede to patients' requests for EC. Patients are therefore not entitled to such aid from pharmacists and are not harmed when pharmacists refuse to give it to them. Neither the antecedent nor the consequent of conditional 2 obtains.

3)   If patients who asked for EC were entitled to get it from some pharmacists, because some (not all) pharmacists have a duty to dispense it, then being refused EC by one of these pharmacists would harm them.

F&L would accept this conditional for the same reasons that they would accept the last one. In addition, they believe that some pharmacists are, or should be, duty-bound to dispense EC. The pharmacists they have in mind are those who work in rural areas or areas where it would be difficult for patients to acquire EC unless some pharmacists were compelled to provide it. There are two parts to F&L's argument here. Part 1 demonstrates that limiting the freedom pharmacists have to turn down potential patients can be legitimate, while Part 2 shows that such limits are appropriate only for some pharmacists.

Part 1 goes as follows: "When individuals confront one another as moral equals, they are not (barring exceptional circumstances) obliged to render more than simple noninterference with the projects of others" (F&L 2005, 585). But pharmacists and their patients are not "moral equals"; rather, one is disadvantaged relative to the other. To explain, the regulatory regime that licenses pharmacists "restricts the liberty of... [patients]"—they cannot go to just anyone for drugs—yet it serves the liberty interests of pharmacists, who are shielded from competition, have greater employment security and income than they otherwise would, and so on (585). Pharmacists have a right to choose their patients, though "some limitation of [this] right...is justifiable compensation to [patients] for having their own domain of choice limited" (585). Thus, out of fairness,[8] pharmacists can be compelled to cooperate with patients who seek services that the pharmacists themselves do not want to provide. The patients may be entitled to these services, in other words, even from pharmacists who object to them.

At the same time, Part 2 has F&L saying that "[p]harmacists' liberty interest in not being compelled to cooperate...with undertakings that they find morally distasteful should not be overridden if potential patients can easily avail themselves of other means for advancing their ends" (588). Thus, when patients could go somewhere else nearby to get EC, they are not entitled to get it from an individual pharmacist and so would not be harmed if one were to turn them away. Pharmacists working in geographical areas where EC is easy to come by therefore do not have a duty to dispense it, while pharmacists who are not in such areas do have this duty.

To summarize F&L's view, in being denied EC *some* patients may be harmed, but not those who could get EC from another pharmacist close by. The latter would be harmed by these refusals only if they faced a true emergency or were entitled to obtain the drug from any pharmacist, yet neither of these conditions holds. Therefore, at most these patients are inconvenienced.

Before analyzing F&L's argument, let me be clear that one could run it with conscientious refusals other than those by pharmacists to EC. For instance, one could argue, following F&L, that many refusals by physicians to perform abortions are merely inconvenient rather than harmful to patients. The reasons are that in many such cases, there is no true emergency, there are other physicians willing to step in to perform the abortion, and the objecting physician does not have a duty to treat, since physicians are free "to choose whom to serve" and they lack a duty to aid. This example demonstrates that F&L's argument generalizes to other typical refusals in reproductive health care.

2. A Harm

In my view, F&L's argument doesn't work, however. They are much too quick in asserting that it is a mere inconvenience for many patients to be denied EC. I will explain why they are unconvincing when they claim that the antecedents of the first two conditionals do not obtain. But first, let me

---

[8] This argument invokes the idea of "fair play," which I discuss in Chapter 5.

introduce another conditional, one allowing that harm to patients from pharmacists denying them EC is common. Since I'm interested in showing that harm to patients is common with other typical refusals as well, I will extend my argument to conscientious refusals to provide abortions by gate-keepers of this service. My argument is broader in this respect than F&L's. I also interpret "harm" differently than they do, while acknowledging that they are not crystal clear on what their own interpretation is. I'll begin by discussing this difference.

F&L appear to be concerned with harms that are also wrongs (i.e., those where people are deprived of that to which they are entitled). There are at least two reasons for this. 1) When F&L discuss harm explicitly,[9] they are responding to the objection that pharmacists should not have the right to refuse to provide EC because these refusals harm patients. But harm to patients would be a reason to deny this right only if the harm were also a wrong. The objector to whom F&L are replying must therefore be using "harm" in this normative sense (Feinberg 1984). To give a viable response, F&L need to prove that there is no normative harm, and so they need to focus on this sort of harm. Thus, it makes sense to assume that when they refer to "harm," they mean normative harm: harm that is also a wrong. 2) F&L do not believe that it is possible for patients who are refused EC to be harmed by this action without being wronged by it.[10] If these patients are not entitled to the drug, then in their view, the objecting pharmacist denies them a benefit but does not harm them.[11]

The first point to make here is that not all harms are wrongs, as I'm sure F&L would agree. To illustrate, I harm you, but do not obviously wrong you, if I cause you grievous injury while warding off a violent attack by you. The "semantic envelope of 'harm'" (to borrow a phrase from F&L 2005, 584) contains more than just states or conditions that are wrongs.[12] I assume that is true in what follows.

---

[9] They do this when they distinguish between failing to benefit people and harming them.

[10] That is true so long as the refusal is a simple one (see note 5). Browbeating by the pharmacist could harm the patient, in F&L's view, although they do not explain why. Presumably, they would say it can interfere with the patient's liberty interests.

[11] F&L have a libertarian view of harm according to which harm results not from failing to provide people with resources to improve their situation or to prevent it from getting worse, but from interfering with their negative liberty. Moreover, the interference must undermine their ability to act freely in the relevant circumstances; it is not enough to erect barriers to their freedom that they can or should be able to surmount. Moral disapproval of their actions would count as such a barrier (F&L 2005, 584).

[12] Philosophers therefore refer to "permissible harm." See, for example, Kamm (2007).

The second point to make is that this semantic envelope as F&L describe it (albeit vaguely) is too narrow. Many of us would include within it circumstances that F&L would summarily exclude: for example, being driven out of business by someone who sets up shop across the street and lures away all of one's customers, or being reduced to tears because someone implies unjustly that one is a reprehensible person. To say that people in situations like these are harmed is perfectly coherent to me, and thus I adopt a broader conception of harm than F&L do. I allow that in doing so, much of what I will say about harm to patients from being refused EC or an abortion will not persuade those who conceive of harm as F&L do.

While "harm" is semantically broader in scope than F&L acknowledge, it is not so broad as to include all forms of disappointment or unpleasantness. Joel Feinberg makes this latter point nicely in his theory of harm. He describes harm in a non-normative sense as a "setback to an interest" (Thomson 1986, 383), where an interest is something in which we have a *stake*, meaning that we are better or worse off depending on the condition of this thing (e.g., our reputation or our family) (Feinberg 1984, 33, 34). People typically do not have a stake in not being disappointed or more generally displeased (Feinberg 1984, 43). For most people, their "psyches are sturdy" enough that they "can take a certain amount of disappointment without [their] interests being affected, that is, without suffering harm" (43).

But not everyone is so sturdy. Moreover, everyone can experience disappointment that is great enough or repeated often enough that it rises to the level of harm in Feinberg's sense (Thomson 1986, 383). Disappointment of this sort interferes, if only temporarily, with one's ability to act in one's interests, because of the mental disturbance or suffering that it causes (Feinberg 1984, 46). An example is disappointment over losing an important contract at work that makes it impossible for one to continue being at work, or disappointment over being told for the hundredth time that one is not as smart as one's brother, which makes one so angry (!) that one cannot concentrate on anything important for a while.

I aim to prove that in all likelihood, the disappointment of being denied EC or similar reproductive services rises to the level of harm for many patients. Whether such harm is normative or non-normative—that is, whether health care professionals also *wrong* patients when they behave in this way—is something I leave open in this chapter.[13] Following Feinberg

---

[13] I *must* leave it open, in fact, if I am to avoid trying to solve the problem of whether these refusals are in fact permissible. Recall, I have the more modest objective of determining what is

(and unless I specify otherwise), I use "harm" to mean a non-normative setback to interests. Moreover, I assume that just as mere disappointment is not harm on Feinberg's theory, mere inconvenience is not harm either. Since something that is a mere inconvenience is only "*slightly* troublesome or difficult" (OED; my emphasis), it alone cannot set an interest back (although repeated inconveniences could do that). Thus, if being denied a service like EC is harmful in Feinberg's sense, then it can't be merely inconvenient.

With this discussion of harm in mind, let me construct another conditional, one—to be clear—in which "harm" does not necessarily mean wrong, as it does in the other conditionals.

4)   If being denied EC by a pharmacist interfered with patients' interests, then this action would harm them.

The antecedent of this conditional probably does obtain for many patients, in part because of the oppressive social structure they inhabit. The cause of the harm may be this structure, not only the pharmacist who refuses to accede to the patient's request. Although harm is not likely to occur in all cases of conscientious refusal to provide EC—presumably, some patients will not mind having to go to another pharmacist—it is likely to occur in many of these cases. The reasons why has to do with the social identities and social experiences of patients.

Let me defend this position, first by linking pharmacists' refusals to oppression and more specifically, to the subjective impact these refusals can have on patients because of how they may be oppressed in society. My claim is not that objecting pharmacists necessarily have oppressive (e.g., sexist) attitudes, but that their refusals could easily reinforce oppression. There are roughly two ways in which this could happen. One is that pharmacists' objections contribute to the stigma many patients experience upon requesting EC. Studies reveal that there is a serious stigma attached to obtaining EC for cisgender women and girls (Shoveller et al. 2007; Wu et al. 2007; Fairhurst et al. 2004; Free et al. 2002), with some studies connecting the stigma directly to social stereotypes about women's sexuality (e.g., Shoveller et al. 2007). The important stereotypes are that women who are sexually

at stake for patients with these refusals (an objective that I pursue as well in Chapter 3). I *will* leave this door open by showing that F&L are not persuasive when they claim that denying patients EC does not "harm" (i.e., wrong) them.

promiscuous are of low character[14]—they are "sluts" or "whores"—and women, more so than men, who have unprotected sex are "irresponsible" or "careless" (Shoveller et al. 2007; Kimport et al. 2011). Stereotypes about the sexuality of minority women are also relevant, including myths about them being promiscuous by nature (e.g., "the lascivious Black woman"; Roberts 1997, 11). In response to stereotypical views about women's sexuality, young women especially worry about being thought of as "that kind of woman" when they ask for EC (Shoveller et al. 2007, 15). Patients requesting EC who do not identify as women could have a similar experience, if despite their gender identity, they have internalized social stereotypes about women, or if similar stereotypes exist for people like them (e.g., bisexual people).[15]

It's not hard to see how conscientious refusals could enhance the stigma that patients feel in requesting EC. After all, the refusals are made on moral grounds by a pharmacist: a respected member of society.[16] In short, these actions can make patients worry more than they otherwise would about being thought of as bad for wanting EC. Objecting pharmacists also need not intend to send such a message for patients to receive it. Actions or statements have meaning against a certain social background (e.g., of myths about women's sexuality); their meaning does not necessarily come from what one intends.

Objecting pharmacists could try to control the meanings their objections have by explaining what grounds them, but it is clear neither that they should be having discussions of this sort with patients, nor that they would succeed regardless in eliminating an oppressive message from their speech.[17] Although they could tell patients who request EC that their concern is not with their sexual behavior, but with the nascent human life that they would

[14] There is a strong link in the public mind between EC and sexual promiscuity. For example, people tend to worry that increased access to EC will increase sexual promiscuity among women (a worry that is unfounded; see Wu et al. 2007).

[15] They may have internalized these stereotypes because now or in the past, they were subject to them as people who presented themselves as, or were interpreted by others to be, women. Note that if they now present as men, however, then they may experience the anti-natalism and transphobia that surround the "pregnant man" (McDonald 2008). If that's true, then their emotional reaction to being denied EC could very well be shock that a health care professional would deny them the means to prevent a pregnancy. The same experience could be had by other patients who routinely experience anti-natalism, such as poor Black women.

[16] Such conduct may be permitted, legally or otherwise, which would probably heighten the stigma surrounding it and the patients' requests for EC. Denying or withdrawing such permission could result in less stigma for patients. I owe this point to an anonymous reviewer from OUP.

[17] Others are more confident than I am that conscientious objectors in health care can issue their objections "without questioning the integrity or moral stature of the patient" (see Lyerly and Little 2013, 261).

jeopardize if they took EC, professionalism probably dictates that they avoid having such conversations with patients (i.e., ones in which they provide unsolicited details about their personal moral beliefs). In giving this explanation for their objection, they might reinforce the patient's oppression anyway. Consider that out of the explanation, a new stereotype about women could rear its head: good women are maternal and do not put the lives of children, especially their own offspring, at risk. Patients who have internalized this stereotype could go from feeling like a whore to feeling like a baby killer, and a female one to boot. Objecting pharmacists might insist, of course, that their concern is not at all with their patients' character: that in no way do they mean to cast aspersions on it. But I suspect that the more they protest, the less convincing and less professional they will be.

Conscientious refusals can contribute to oppression in a further way, one that applies to circumstances where the refusals are legally (or otherwise) permitted and where the patients are not necessarily concerned with how their request for EC might influence people's thoughts about their sexuality, their degree of moral responsibility, or their maternal instincts. That they live in a society that allows pharmacists—the gatekeepers to EC—to deny people this drug could confirm to patients, along with other factors perhaps (such as inadequate protection from sexual assault and poor access to abortion services), that their society does not respect them. It does not value their ability to govern their bodies or their lives. The subjective impact of conscientious refusals on patients who feel such disrespect will be severe. They are also probably large in number, assuming that many patients who request EC feel entitled, on some level, to get it.[18]

To summarize, pharmacists' refusals to dispense EC reinforce oppression when they contribute to the stigma that often accompanies a request for EC and also to the sense of many patients who make these requests that their society does not respect them. Notice that other typical refusals can have many of the same effects. That is particularly true of physician refusals to provide patients with abortions, because of the status physicians have as respected members of society and as the sole gatekeepers to abortion in many contexts,[19] but also because for many patients, there is serious stigma

---

[18] Evidence of this feeling comes from a study showing that overall, American women strongly oppose the right of pharmacists and other health professionals to refuse out of conscience to provide them with reproductive services (Miller 2000).

[19] That is true—physicians are the sole gatekeepers—despite recommendations to the contrary by the World Health Organization (2015). It is also increasingly not the case with respect to medical abortions (Kapp et al. 2017).

attached to seeking an abortion (see Chapter 3), just as there is with requesting EC. In fact, the two sorts of stigma overlap substantially because they are informed by some of the same stereotypes, including that women who have unprotected sex are "loose" or "irresponsible." Keeping this in mind in what follows allows us to see how much of my analysis of pharmacists' refusals to dispense EC applies equally well to conscientious refusals to provide abortions.

Having explored the connection between conscientious refusals and oppression, we can now understand which interests of patients are "set back" when they are refused EC, and therefore why many patients can be harmed by these refusals. These interests include patients' autonomy in obtaining EC (their reproductive autonomy), their moral identity (as a good or fine person), and the sense of security that goes along with living in a society that respects them. Regardless of the moral stance one takes on EC, I assume one can agree that these are genuine interests and that setting them back is indeed harmful, if not wrongful.

Conscientious refusals threaten patients' reproductive autonomy if they enhance the stigma associated with EC so much that out of shame or embarrassment, the patients stop trying to acquire EC (Stein 2005; Shoveller et al. 2007). Empirical evidence suggests that the stigma alone is enough to prevent some patients from ever asking for this drug. For them, it is easier "not to think about the risk of pregnancy, which might not occur, than to endure the stigmatization over the need for [EC]" (Free et al. 2002, 1394, 1395). Other patients who fear being stigmatized overcome this feeling to ask for EC. But would they keep trying to get it after being refused it for moral reasons—and by a health professional? To soldier on would presumably require more bravery and self-assurance than some patients can muster, particularly those who feel the stigma intensely because of their age or who are stigmatized more than others because of their minority status. Put simply, conscientious refusals will deter some patients—granted, perhaps only a small number of them—from accessing EC, because of the stigma attached to doing so. These patients will be harmed in not being able to exercise their reproductive autonomy. Of course, the impact on their autonomy will be especially severe if they get pregnant because of not taking EC and have to have an abortion or suffer through a "forced gestation" (Little 1999).

Alternatively, or in addition, conscientious refusals can set back the interest patients have in maintaining their moral identity. The refusals have this effect when they trigger in patients' minds oppressive norms that they have internalized and that vilify them or their behavior. The mental image brought on by the refusal of them having a low character could linger despite their best efforts to erase it. Moreover, if it does linger, then their hold on their moral identity as a different kind of person—a responsible kind—has loosened. We do have reports of patients feeling humiliated, like they had to defend what kind of person they are, when they were refused EC.[20] Being humiliated—or "branded a moral transgressor" (F&L 2005, 583)—is harmful in Feinberg's sense if it damages something in which one has a stake. I conjecture that what is at stake for some patients when they are refused EC is a continuous grip on their moral identity,[21] and that oppressive norms help to explain why that is the case.

Finally, conscientious refusals—coupled with legal (or other societal) permission of them—put patients' sense of security at risk when they confirm to them that their society does not respect their ability to govern their body. To sense disrespect of this sort from whoever is in power is to feel vulnerable. People clearly have an interest in not feeling this way, but rather in being secure in knowing that their society respects their bodily integrity. Conscientious refusals that violate this interest harm patients.

I assume that for many patients, refusals to provide them with EC will set back at least one of the above interests: in their reproductive autonomy, their moral identity, or their sense of security. And as a result, many patients will be harmed by these refusals. What is at stake for them in being denied EC is the avoidance of harm, rather than mere inconvenience. It should be clear that conscientious refusals to abortion by gatekeepers of it can have the very same effects. Essentially, by enhancing abortion stigma and not allowing patients to control what happens to their bodies, these refusals threaten the interests I have identified.

It should also be clear that the harm I've discussed will occur regardless of whether the patients can access the service they seek somewhere else close by. Indeed, I assumed that they had this level of access to EC when describing how refusals to dispense it can interfere with patients' autonomy, moral identity, or sense of security. Such disruption occurred in the scenarios I used because of the experience of a refusal, not because of a lack of access.[22]

---

[20] See, for example, Gee (2006) and Lucero II (2018).

[21] Interestingly, some bioethicists give the same answer to what is at stake for conscientious objectors in being denied the ability to object: namely, their moral identity (see Wicclair 2011; 2017, and Chapter 1).

[22] I accept that if objectors could refuse to dispense EC without ever interacting with individual patients who request it and the patients can still obtain EC, then the refusals would not be harmful. I consider ways of avoiding these interactions, and whether measures to avoid them are morally permissible, in Chapter 6.

Let me briefly address two further issues about harm to patients from conscientious refusals to provide EC. First, would the harm exist in the absence of oppression? I doubt it, mainly because in such a society, a moral objection to a patient requesting EC would not have the same social meaning as it does in our society. It could not reinforce in patients' minds the harmful message that they are careless sluts or second-class citizens, for example. Perhaps there would still be stigma associated with EC—that is, gender-neutral stigma about being irresponsible with contraception—but presumably it would be weaker than the stigma we have now, and patients would be better able to cope with it and prevent it, along with the pharmacist's objection, from setting their interests back, simply because they would be more empowered. But I speculate and do so too freely perhaps. I prefer to concentrate on actual patients, who suffer, generally speaking, from the kinds of oppression I've identified.

Second, are there ways, other than those I've considered, that conscientious refusals to provide EC could violate patients' interests and consequently harm them? The answer is yes, since the refusals can damage patients' interests in general by making them so angry that they are distracted from doing what is important to them. The experience of conscientious refusal can also amount to betrayal—one's trust in one's health care professional is betrayed—which itself is harmful. I discuss matters of trust, betrayal, and conscientious refusal in Chapter 3. Aside from the harm that is associated with them, I assume I have covered in this chapter the most serious ways in which conscientious refusals can harm patients.

Although harm to the above interests—in reproductive autonomy, a moral identity, and a sense of security—is serious, it may nevertheless be morally permissible, as I alluded to earlier. In other words, pharmacists may do nothing morally wrong in causing this harm. Whether that is true will depend on whether they have a right to conscientious objection that trumps the protection of these interests.[23]

Some people will want to insist that the harm I've discussed is simply irrelevant to the debate over a pharmacist's right of conscience. They will point to the fact that objecting pharmacists are not the sole and perhaps not even the main cause of this harm. Surely, we shouldn't impose restrictions

---

[23] Whether it is true *could* also depend on whether the moral views that inform their conscience are correct: that is, whether, despite the harm to patients in being refused access to EC, access to it is morally impermissible. The correctness of objectors' moral views does not shape the moral permissibility of their actions, according to the theory I defend in this book, although I did support such a view in the past (McLeod 2008; see also Ben-Moshe 2019).

on pharmacists' right to conscience because of harm caused by stereotypes that pharmacists themselves may not even accept! My response to this objection is twofold. First, it is not obvious that restricting the behavior of health care professionals for these reasons is illegitimate. It seems plausible that as part of their larger duty to respect patient autonomy, these professionals have a duty to do what they can to counteract harmful effects that stereotypes can have on patient autonomy (McLeod 2002). I return to this issue in Chapter 5.[24]

Second, if we ignore the kind of harm I've discussed, as F&L do, then we fail to deal with the conflict between the objecting pharmacist and the patient as it actually exists: as a conflict between two people who are morally unequal not simply because the pharmacist is privileged by a licensing scheme, but also because the patient is often an oppressed person in society. F&L write, "pharmacist and prospective [patient] do not stand to each other as any two random agents endeavoring to secure their various ends as they make their way through the world" (585). They assume that is true in cases where the prospective patient is seeking EC only because one of the "two random agents" is a pharmacist. But surely it is true as well because one of them is likely oppressed (as a woman, a trans person, a woman of color, etc.). We appreciate this fact, moreover, only by attending to how conscientious refusals to EC can harm patients as members of social groups.

In general, once we situate conscientious refusals to EC within their social context, it becomes plausible to believe, regardless of whether EC is readily available elsewhere, that for many patients, the effect of these refusals is harm rather than mere inconvenience. F&L fail to see the harm not only because they conceive of harm too narrowly in their discussion, but also because in analyzing these refusals, they take them out of a social context of oppression. People who view physician refusals to provide abortions as a mere inconvenience to patients make the same mistake. The conclusions I have drawn about pharmacist refusals generalize to these other objections, because of similarities in what it means to be denied EC or an abortion on moral grounds, as a member of an oppressed group, and by a health care professional.

I have said I want to leave open whether the harm to patients from pharmacist refusals is normative (i.e., a wrong). If F&L are correct, however,

---

[24] And to put the point in terms of language from that chapter, health care professionals have a duty to attend to the circumstantial vulnerability of patients that is brought about by their oppression.

that no individual pharmacist has a duty to dispense EC to patients who could easily get it elsewhere, then by refusing to give EC to these patients, pharmacists do not wrong them; whatever harm the patients might suffer could not be a wrong. So, let me end by showing that F&L are not convincing when they make this claim, and are therefore not convincing when they suggest that refusals cannot wrong patients who have other means of obtaining EC. Individual pharmacists could indeed have the duty to dispense EC in these cases. To be clear, rather than argue for this view here, I will simply show that it is plausible and in doing so, will cast doubt on the truth of F&L's position on the duty to dispense.

3. *Emergency* Contraception?

Recall the first conditional:

1) If patients who requested EC faced a true emergency, then being refused it by a pharmacist would harm them.

F&L suggest that while emergencies are "measured in minutes,"[25] "women have up to 72 hours after unprotected intercourse to secure medicine to block pregnancy" (2005, 582). Yet even if the timing were tighter than that, F&L would say we cannot insist on "emergency" as the appropriate label, because it implies that unwanted pregnancies are a serious problem.[26] How we ought to characterize these pregnancies is again "precisely the crux of the parties' dispute" (582). F&L therefore state that we cannot legitimately claim obtaining EC is an emergency for patients who request it.

This argument is unconvincing, however. First, EC's "contraceptive efficacy decreases dramatically during [the] seventy-two hour window" (Davidoff 2006, 20); the drug is most effective if used 12–24 hours after unprotected intercourse (Greenberger and Vogelstein 2005). "[E]ffective contraceptive relief is [still] not measured in minutes" (F&L 2005, 582), although it is measured in hours and the relevant hours may be small in number. I am not

---

[25] "Unlike someone in cardiac arrest or lying by the side of the road with a spurting artery, effective contraceptive relief is not measured in minutes" (F&L 2005, 582).

[26] The assumption here is that emergencies exist only when *immediate* action is necessary to avert a situation that is *serious* (OED). I would modify this definition as follows: emergencies exist when prudence dictates that we engage in immediate action to avert a situation that is serious.

at all persuaded that emergencies must be measured in minutes rather than hours (or even days). If we knew that a bomb was set to go off in a public place in 72 hours, then we would clearly have an emergency on our hands.

Second, if we accept along with F&L that averting an unwanted pregnancy could not be an emergency, then are we not taking the perspective of the objecting pharmacist, rather than being neutral between the pharmacist and the patient? I do not see how we can be neutral, given that we are faced with two discrete alternatives: either EC is *emergency* contraception or it is not. We could also take sides on this issue without settling the matter of whether pharmacists can ever refuse to dispense EC (which, again, is not something I want to do in this chapter). They could still refuse, in some circumstances at least, if avoiding an unwanted pregnancy were an emergency; they could do it when there is a back-up pharmacist in place who could deal with the emergency at hand (Wicclair 2006, 239; see also Chapter 6).[27]

Let me review why the risk of unwanted pregnancy is often serious enough that it could be an emergency for patients if they have only 72 hours to stave it off. Pregnancy can jeopardize patients' lives, their physical or mental health, or their entire future as they envision it. Pregnancy endangers the life of patients with certain health conditions (Greenberger and Vogelstein 2005, 1557; Lyerly and Little 2013); for some, it represents a "period of risk" for physical abuse by husbands or partners (Saltzman et al. 2003); it jeopardizes the mental health of patients who are pregnant due to rape and who experience the pregnancy as a nine-month continuation of that rape; it ruins the future plans of many patients, who know they could not go through the intimacy of gestation (Little 1999) and then relinquish their child for adoption, and who also realize they will be the child's primary caretaker; and for some, it means that they will be dependent on a partner who treats them badly. It follows that for many patients, what is at stake with an unwanted pregnancy is nothing short of life, health, freedom, and/or respect. Given how essential these goods are, should we not conclude, when people have up to 72 hours to avoid the loss of them, that they face a true emergency?[28]

---

[27] I am open to this possibility, at least in cases where there is *not* an existing relationship between the patient and the pharmacist (see Chapter 5). That said, I generally believe that conscientious objectors have a duty to treat in emergencies.

[28] To be clear, I do not mean to suggest here that needing an abortion, as opposed to EC, would normally count as an emergency. That wouldn't be true according the conception of an emergency that underlies much of what I say above: that an emergency exists when prudence dictates that we engage in immediate action to avert a situation that is serious (see note 84). Using this definition, we can conclude that needing an abortion is often not an emergency. It is not when *immediate* action is unnecessary, because it will not make a significant difference to

Still, some people will object to the idea that an unwanted pregnancy is so terrible that a substantial risk of one occurring counts as an emergency. What about the "nascent human life" that could flourish if the pregnancy were allowed to proceed? Or what about the possibility of the patient having an abortion? I will evaluate these points, but only briefly, since again my purpose is to show just that F&L's view is unpersuasive, not that the opposite view is correct. The pharmacist who is opposed to EC believes that a nascent human life could be "in dire jeopardy" (F&L 2005, 582).[29] Even assuming that is true, however, unlike the patient requesting EC, the embryo does not have a personal future that is at stake with the decision of whether to dispense EC (McInerney 1990). Furthermore, its life is completely dependent on another's and will continue to be so (if it survives) for months or years; we cannot simply choose its life or its future over that of the patient. Thus, even if EC threatened a nascent human life, it could still be an emergency for patients to obtain EC.

What about the objection that patients could simply have an abortion if they get pregnant after not being able to access EC? This suggestion—to put it mildly—is distasteful. The decision to terminate a pregnancy is emotionally difficult for many patients (Joffe 2013; Macfarlane 2008). Also, abortion is not readily available for many of them,[30] it is out of the question for some, and in any case, it is painful, particularly if it involves surgery.[31] To imply, as F&L do, that there is no emergency because "subsequent abortion is

---

the patient's welfare. In other words, it will not make a significant difference whether the abortion occurs one or two weeks after the initial request for it rather than happening right way.

[29] The literature mentions two ways in which EC could jeopardize the life of this entity: 1) by terminating a pregnancy; or 2) by preventing the implantation of a fertilized egg. There is no evidence that currently available forms of EC (i.e., Plan B and similar hormonal regimens) interfere with an established pregnancy (Card 2007, 10; Schulz et al. 2016). And there is some controversy over whether they can have postfertilization effects; for example, Card cites evidence to the contrary (2007 11; citing Croxatto et al. 2004, see also Gemzell-Danielsson et al. 2014), while Baergen and Owens (PharmD) claim that "available data on Plan B do not rule out the possibility of a postfertilization mechanism of action" (2006, 1279). Indeed, some argue (in Catholic journals) that its primary mechanism of action is to prevent implantation (e.g., Peck et al. 2016).

[30] For example, in Canada there are significant barriers to accessing surgical abortions; as of 2006, only 15.9 percent of Canadian hospitals provided this service (Shaw 2006). The recent approval of the abortion pill Mifepristone provides hope that access to abortions in general will increase across the country (http://www.nafcanada.org/access-abortion-ca.html (retrieved June 9, 2019); Dunn and Brooks 2018).

[31] An abortion can be medical (involving the abortion pill) or surgical. Many patients liken the experience of a medical abortion to having an early miscarriage, which suggests that a medical abortion could also be physically painful. See https://www.plannedparenthood.org/learn/abortion/the-abortion-pill/how-does-the-abortion-pill-work (retrieved June 9, 2019).

available" to patients who cannot get EC is to fail to understand what it means to contemplate an abortion (2005, 582). It also fails to appreciate that emergencies can exist even when there is only a chance of something bad happening. A small house fire is an emergency, for example. To question this by saying that the house may not burn down, and that even if it does, one could rebuild at a later date, is ludicrous. Similarly, to insist that being at risk for an unwanted pregnancy is not an emergency because the pregnancy may not occur, and even if it does, the patient could have an abortion, is absurd.

For these reasons, I remain unconvinced that patients requesting EC are not in an emergency situation and that pharmacists do not have a duty to dispense EC as part of their larger duty to provide care in emergencies. Pharmacists could very well have this duty, which means that the harm caused by pharmacists' refusals to provide patients with EC could very well be a wrong.

4. A Duty to Dispense?

Recall the second conditional:

2)   If patients who sought EC were entitled to get it from any pharmacist, because every pharmacist had a duty to dispense EC to any patient who makes a legitimate request for it, then being refused EC by a pharmacist would harm them.

F&L's main reason for rejecting the duty mentioned here is that, like other professionals, pharmacists have the freedom to choose whom to serve. F&L take this freedom to be so extensive that it eliminates the possibility that many pharmacists have a duty to dispense. I believe this view is implausible for reasons I discuss in Chapters 5 and 6 and will briefly outline here.

According to F&L's interpretation of the freedom to choose whom to serve, professionals can "turn down potential [patients] with whom they feel uncomfortable working either for moral or other reasons" (2005, 582). One thing to highlight about this statement is that it concerns the freedom to choose whether to serve *prospective* patients rather than actual ones, meaning people with whom the pharmacist has a prior relationship as *their* pharmacist. (The freedom to choose whom to serve normally focuses on interactions with prospective patients; see Chapter 6.) F&L ignore the possibility that some requests for EC come from *actual* patients, in which case the pharmacist could have a fiduciary duty to prioritize the patients' interests over the pharmacist's own and ultimately to dispense EC to them. I develop this "prioritizing approach" in Chapter 5. Here, I simply want to flag that pharmacists could indeed have a duty to dispense EC if the patient requesting it was their own. Let me concentrate in what follows on cases where the patient is a prospective one.

F&L's understanding of the freedom to choose whom to serve is too broad if there are reasons for rejecting prospective patients that are simply out of bounds for health care professionals (Arras 1988, 15). Would it be appropriate, for example, if, out of moral indifference to unhealthy people and a concern for their own lifestyle, some family physicians refused to take on new patients who are unhealthy and whom they feel would take up too much of their time?[32] Many of us would say no, presumably because we believe that moral indifference and pure self-interest are not legitimate reasons for health care professionals to turn away prospective patients. And if we're right, then these professionals have an obligation that precludes them from rejecting patients for these reasons. John Arras claims that they have a "role-specific duty to care for the vulnerable"—people who are vulnerable, presumably, because of their health status (1988, 15; see also Clark 2005; Wicclair 2006; Card 2007). I propose instead (in Chapter 6) that many health care professionals have a duty to the public to promote equitable access to care and public health. Importantly, the relevant duty, in my theory and Arras's, constrains the freedom health care professionals have to choose whom to serve.

Let me be clear that Arras and I claim not that health care professionals should have no freedom to choose their patients, but rather that any such freedom should be tempered by a duty either to care for the medically vulnerable, which is Arras's view, or to promote equitable access to care and public health, which is my view. In deciding whether to heed the requests of prospective patients for services, health care professionals need to consider whether turning the patients down would violate a duty of this sort. It's possible that denying their requests would be morally appropriate, since the duty itself could require that health care professionals refuse some requested services (i.e., those that would be harmful in the circumstances). Alternatively, concern for the medically vulnerable or for equitable access to care could

---

[32] This practice—of refusing patients with complex medical problems and choosing those who are relatively healthy—has been called the "cherry picking" of patients (Milne et al. 2014).

legitimately be overridden by other concerns (though presumably only moral ones, including perhaps the professional's own conscience).

Overall, Arras and I demonstrate, contra F&L, that pharmacists' freedom to choose whom to serve could be quite narrow. That is true no matter whether the pharmacists are one among many in a 1-mile radius or the only pharmacist in a 100-mile radius. Pharmacists could very well have an obligation to dispense EC, in other words, even to patients who could easily get it somewhere else. Similarly, physicians or other health care professionals could have a duty to treat patients who request abortions. The duty to dispense or to treat could be part of a larger duty either to care for the medically vulnerable or to promote equitable access to care and public health. Alternatively, it could exist on the grounds that having access to contraception or abortion and being spared the harm of being refused it are central to patients' welfare. Regardless of its origins, however, with this duty in place, the moral situation of individual conscientious objectors is more complicated than F&L make it out to be. They would be in a moral conflict situation, rather than merely a situation of having a certain desire and deciding how to act on it.

5. Conclusion

What the moral situation actually is of individual objectors is determined not just by their moral duties but also by what is at stake for patients in being denied standard reproductive health services. I have argued that what is at stake for many patients in being refused EC is their reproductive autonomy, their moral identity, their sense of security, or all of the above. What is more, this argument generalizes to other typical refusals in reproductive health care, including refusals to provide abortions. It is therefore reasonable to conclude, based on a plausible conception of harm, that patients who experience these denials of service are harmed rather than merely inconvenienced. What they undergo is no small matter, morally speaking.

3

Damage to Trust

When patients experience the kinds of conscientious refusals that are typical in reproductive health care, what is the likely impact on them? According to Chapter 2, the answer lies in *harm* in the form of some loss of reproductive autonomy, of a moral identity as a good or fine person, or of a sense of security. The focus there was primarily on conscientious refusals by pharmacists to provide emergency contraception. Because of the stigma for patients surrounding requests for EC, having them denied by pharmacists on grounds of conscience can cause such humiliation that patients stop their search for EC or have their moral identity—as a good or fine person—shaken. As well, because of how important it is for patients to be able to avoid unwanted pregnancies, discovering that pharmacists have the right to conscientiously refuse them EC (i.e., where they have this right), can undermine any security the patients have in knowing that they can control what happens to their body. This argument about harm to patients from conscientious refusals has a wider relevance than pharmacist refusals to offer EC. In Chapter 2, I demonstrated how the argument extends, in particular, to refusals by physicians to provide abortions.

Chapter 2 did not describe all of the ways in which conscientious refusals can harm patients, however. Another way that they can cause harm is by damaging the trust that patients have in health care professionals and health care professions.[1] Damage to trust can occur through discovering that one's trust has been betrayed, been let down, or was simply misplaced. Drawing on the account of harm discussed in Chapter 2, we can say that such occurrences are harmful if they set one's interests back. I assume in the present chapter that patients have strong interests in being able to trust health care professionals and professions, generally speaking.[2] They also often have an interest in maintaining existing relationships with particular health care

---

[1] Trust in the profession can be understood as trust in the relevant professional organization or in those who direct this organization.

[2] That is true mainly because of their vulnerability in seeking out good health care. On the value of patient trust, see O'Neill (2002), Clark (2002), Pellegrino (1991), and Whitbeck (1995).

Conscience in Reproductive Health Care: Prioritizing Patient Interests. Carolyn McLeod, Oxford University Press (2020).
© Carolyn McLeod.
DOI: 10.1093/oso/9780198732723.001.0001

professionals, those with whom they've felt comfortable, who know their health history, who perhaps are excellent diagnosticians, or who may be the only health care professional of their kind that the patient can access. These precious relationships will not continue—or at least will not continue to be effective—without trust. Thus, if conscientious refusals damage the trust of patients, then they will be harmful. I argue in this chapter that these refusals can, and indeed most likely will, have this effect.

It is important to minimize the damage that conscientious refusals cause to patient trust, because of how valuable trust is for effective patient–health care professional relationships; some loss of trust from these refusals may be unavoidable, however, while the resulting harm itself is morally permissible. I do not take a stand in this chapter on whether harm of this sort would be permissible, just as I did not take a stand on whether the harm discussed in Chapter 2 was permissible. It may be that conscientious refusals themselves are permissible and thus so is the damage they inevitably cause to patient trust. Rather than focus on this issue here, I do two things. First, I aim to show that trust is among the interests at stake for patients in allowing health care professionals to make conscientious refusals. Second, I critique a response to this concern about trust by Holly Fernandez Lynch in her *Conflicts of Conscience in Health Care* (2008).

Lynch develops what she calls an "institutional compromise" to the conflicts that conscientious refusals generate. She believes one benefit of her solution to these disputes is that it would enhance trust between health care professionals and patients, and prevent damage to trust from conscientious refusals (90). I will endeavor to show, on the contrary, that insofar as our concern is with patient trust, we should reject Lynch's proposal. I will also describe briefly the type of proposal that we should endorse instead, which is one that aligns with the prioritizing approach to conscientious refusals that I defend in Chapters 5 and 6.

Like Chapter 2, this one uses examples throughout of a particular kind of typical refusal in reproductive health care: namely, a refusal by a physician to provide abortion services. The reasons for the focus on physicians include the fact that Lynch does the same and that in many jurisdictions, physicians are the sole gatekeepers to abortion services.[3] I concentrate on abortion for two reasons, one being that paradigm cases of conscientious refusal in

---

[3] See Chapter 2, note 77. In other jurisdictions, other health care professionals, such as midwives and nurse practitioners, are permitted to provide these services and may indeed be the sole providers of them. See, e.g., Weitz et al. (2013) and Holcombe et al. (2015).

health care (not just reproductive health care) involve abortion.[4] The other reason concerns the relative wealth of empirical evidence available about people's abortion experiences, evidence that brings into stark relief what is at stake with regard to patient trust in allowing health care professionals to make conscientious refusals. Like in Chapter 2, the discussion in this chapter will have implications beyond the specific type of examples I give to other typical refusals in reproductive health care, including those by pharmacists to offer services like EC. (I will point out how the argument extends to these other refusals, when it is not obvious how it does so.) My overall goal is to build on our understanding of the harm to patients that occurs when health care professionals make typical conscientious refusals.

1. The Damage

Conscientious objections will often seriously damage patients' trust in the objectors themselves, but they can also impair their trust in the objectors' health care professions and in other members of them. This is my claim in this section. It is significant that the damage can extend beyond trust in the objector, because otherwise it would be limited to a relationship that may end abruptly after the objection occurs. Most patients would seek out a different health care professional if they felt they could no longer trust their own, although, of course, not all patients have this luxury. (Those who do not include many patients who are poor, live in rural areas, and cannot afford to travel to see a different professional.) That conscientious objections jeopardize trust in objectors is itself a serious concern, but so is their potential to interfere with patient trust more broadly.

Different features of trust are relevant to understanding how and why patients trust health care professionals and the damage that conscientious objections can do to their trust. In outlining these features, I will draw on my previous work on trust (McLeod 2002; 2015) and on the work of others, particularly Annette Baier, whose theory of trust has been influential.[5] As I will discuss, her framework is also especially helpful in describing the

---

[4] Some say that they are the most prevalent form of conscientious refusal (IWHC 2017).
[5] It has been influential in philosophy (see my *Stanford Encyclopedia of Philosophy* entry on trust, McLeod 2015), in bioethics (see, e.g., Pellegrino and Thomasma 1993 and O'Neill 2002), and in law, especially fiduciary law (see, e.g., Fox-Decent 2005).

basic elements of the trust that patients have (or can have) in health care professionals.

In addition, I will highlight an element of trust that I've defended in the past but that is missing from prominent philosophical theories on the subject, including Baier's: that in trusting others, we expect that they will share, or be committed to, enough of our values that we can indeed trust them in the domain(s) of our interactions with them. Discussing this expectation is important for different reasons, one being that Lynch relies on it substantially (though only implicitly) in her theory about how to remedy the damage to patient trust that conscientious refusals can cause. Another reason is that the expectation helps to explain why the solution I provide to the problem of conscientious refusals (i.e., in Chapters 5 and 6) is justifiable and also preferable to Lynch's solution in terms of how well it supports patient trust. Lastly, and most importantly, it is simply true that an expectation about having some shared values is a key feature of many trust relationships, and theories of trust that do not acknowledge this fact are inadequate.[6]

The following are the features of trust that I'll discuss and will claim can be undermined by conscientious refusals: (a) reliance on the competence of the trustee (i.e., the one trusted), (b) reliance on the goodwill of the trustee, and (c) an expectation about some shared values. The idea is that conscientious objection can stop patients from having (a), (b), or (c) entirely or to some degree, and therefore can destroy or diminish their trust. To be clear about these features, they may only be common to many instances of trust rather than being necessary for trust.[7] They also, together, may not be sufficient for trust. To be sure, there are important elements of trust that are missing from this list. Examples are the vulnerability of the truster to the trustee and the discretionary power of trustees—that is, the power they have to use their discretion to decide how to live up to the trust that is placed in them (see Baier 1986, esp. 237–9). I assume these features are intimately bound up with (a)–(c), such that they (the vulnerability and the power)

---

[6] Not all of these theories are subject to this criticism. Some (other than mine; McLeod 2002) include an expectation about shared values, norms, or rules. See Mullin (2005), Smith (2008), and Lahno (2001).

[7] Following Brennan Jacoby (2011), I accept that trust is a cluster concept (and argued for something similar in my book on trust; 2002). In other words, in my view, what Natalie Stoljar says about the concept "woman" is also true about "trust": "there is a cluster of different features in our concept of woman and in order for an individual to satisfy the concept, it is sufficient (and necessary) to satisfy *enough* of, rather than all and only, the features in the cluster" (Stoljar 2011, 42). The features of trust that I identify here are part of the cluster that makes up our concept of trust.

would decline along with the inability of the truster to continue relying on the goodwill or competence of the trustee, or expecting that the two had some shared values. Thus, leaving them off the above list is not a problem.

Features (a)–(c) are not sufficient even to describe the effects that conscientious refusals can have on trust, since what Baier calls the "climate of trust" is also significant (1986, 245).[8] More specifically, norms informing the social climate that concern the trustworthiness of health care professionals and of patients are relevant. These aspects of climate influence whether (a)–(c) are present in the first place, but also how damaging conscientious refusals can be to them, or so I will argue.

Let me go through (a)–(c) in turn. Using, again, examples involving physicians and abortion, I will describe how social climate affects each of these features of trust, how conscientious refusals threaten each of them, and why none on their own can explain the damage that conscientious refusals can do. Since I will be focusing on how conscientious refusals can jeopardize patient trust, I will be using scenarios that involve patients who trust their physician and the medical profession initially, but who then have their trust compromised by a refusal from their physician. Conscientious refusals can also exacerbate existing distrust among patients who had little trust in health care professionals or professions to begin with.[9] While this concern is certainly important, I will concentrate on the effects of these refusals on *trust*.

1.1 Reliance on Competence

There is general agreement in the literature on trust that an important element of trust is reliance in (or optimism about)[10] the competence of trustees to

---

[8] This climate, as she describes it, includes norms and conventions (e.g., about promising) that make it relatively easy for people to trust one another. They allow people to have "a presumption of a sort of trustworthiness" in one another (Baier 1986, 246). The relevant norms extend to what we expect of people in certain social roles, such as that of a physician (245). Baier emphasizes that the norms and conventions that make up a climate of trust can be oppressive. She says, for instance, "the right to make promises and the power to have one's promises accepted are not possessed by everyone in relation to everyone else" (e.g., by slaves in relation to free persons; 246). Consequently, the convention of promise keeping will facilitate not only trust but also distrust (e.g., in those who lack the power to make promises in a trustworthy manner). The climate of trust will be more like a climate of trust and *distrust*, which is a point that Baier does not make clear. I make use of these features of the climate of "trust" below.

[9] Such distrust can be a serious problem among African Americans in the United States, for example. See, e.g., Almassi (2014) and Tweedy (2015).

[10] See Jones (1996) and McGeer (2008).

do what one trusts them to do. It is clear that most trust would not exist without this feature.[11] Patients would not trust physicians to supply them with abortion services, for example, if they knew they could not rely on the physicians being competent to do so (i.e., having knowledge of these services and how to provide them). Moreover, if patients do trust particular physicians in this regard, without knowing of *them* that they possess the relevant competence, then the trust must occur because of a climate of trust surrounding physicians, one that includes norms about them being clinically competent to care for patients who choose to have an abortion or request any standard health care service. The same sort of reasoning applies to other health care professionals; patients would not trust a pharmacist's advice about the use of EC, for instance, if they did not think that the pharmacist, or pharmacists in general, were experts on EC.

Consider first how conscientious refusals can interfere with the ability of patients to rely on the competence of objectors, and second, how this problem can affect their trust in the objector's profession and in other members of it. Conscientious refusals can damage trust in objectors by revealing to patients that the objector lacks competence or certain competencies. Depending, perhaps, on how objectors express their refusals, patients' trust in their competence will likely decrease. Imagine conscientiously objecting physicians who add to their moral complaint about abortion a concern—often uttered by anti-abortionists—that abortion jeopardizes patients' health (by, e.g., causing breast cancer or depression).[12] This claim, which is false, will confirm in the mind of patients who know the truth about these matters that the objectors are simply not competent medically when it comes to abortion.

Alternatively, some objectors will not misconstrue the effects of an abortion yet will not be competent to provide abortions, because they conscientiously refused training in abortion services. Where such training is mandatory (e.g., for OB-GYNs), conscientious objectors can usually (not always) opt out of it (see Osnos 2002; Laurance 2007; Downie and Nassar 2008; Fiala et al. 2016). Those who can and do opt out will then have to turn

---

[11] To note one exception, consider what philosophers call "therapeutic trust" (Horsburgh 1960), where one trusts someone with the hope of engendering greater trustworthiness in that person (e.g., a child). Such an attitude involves little if any reliance on, as opposed to hopefulness about, the competence of the other (McGeer 2008).

[12] See, e.g., the Campaign Life Coalition's website on harm to patients from abortion: http://www.campaignlifecoalition.com/index.php?p=Harm_to_Women (retrieved May 16, 2019). For criticism of claims about a risk of breast cancer, see Planned Parenthood (2013), and of claims about depression, see Weitz et al. (2008, 87).

down requests for abortions in their practice, because they lack the requisite technical competence. Since their incompetence is deliberate, however, and exists because of a conscientious objection, their refusal arguably counts as such an objection. Moreover, it presents another scenario in which conscientious refusals to provide standard services can undermine patient trust in the competence of physicians. (And of course, opportunities to conscientiously refuse to obtain health professional education for other health care professionals, such as pharmacists, would have the same effect.)[13]

A further kind of scenario is one in which objectors treat patients who ask for an abortion so shabbily—without an ounce of sympathy, for example— that the objectors show that they lack the *moral* competence needed to care for patients in this context and are not trustworthy in this regard.[14] "Moral competence" refers to the skills needed to understand and fulfill one's moral responsibilities (Jones 1996, 7). Someone who is morally incompetent is simply not capable of being morally responsible. Reliance on competence within a trust relationship can target moral or non-moral competence or both (Jones 1996).

In all three of the scenarios above, the conscientious objection undermines the patients' reliance on the objectors' competence to provide abortion services. Yet notice how easily the objections could have a wider impact on how the patients view the objectors' competence. The patients might wonder what else the objectors are not competent to do, other than serve patients who request abortions. What other medical facts are they inclined to be mistaken about because of their moral beliefs? What other training did they refuse to acquire or not take seriously as a student? In what other situations will they demonstrate a lack of moral competence? Given what is normally at stake in medical encounters, patients are likely to be cautious about relying on physicians' competence in general after witnessing their incompetence in a specific area. My point is not that patients *should* be reluctant to display such widespread reliance, but only that they may do so and their trust in these physicians would suffer as a result.

---

[13] An example of such an opportunity exists in Canada, where training for pharmacists in dispensing the abortion pill is not mandatory (MacKinnon 2017).

[14] Jessica Shaw gives a relevant and stark example involving a patient who requested a referral for an abortion from her physician, who in turn "placed a stethoscope on her abdomen and said, "I love you mommy... I love you mommy..." in rhythm with her heartbeat" (2006, 48; cited in Shaw 2013, 12). The physician could, and indeed should, have convinced the patient that he was morally incompetent by engaging in such manipulation.

A conscientious objection that negatively disrupts patients' reliance on the competence of objectors can also negatively affect their trust in the objectors' profession and in other similar professionals. Many patients will question how the profession could allow its members to practice in this way, without the requisite technical or moral knowledge of how to care for patients properly.[15] In particular, how could it permit that some of its members not learn how to perform a procedure—abortion—that can be lifesaving in some instances and that some of their patients will most likely need? How could it allow some of them to perpetuate myths about the health effects of standard procedures (e.g., abortion) or show little compassion toward patients who request them? The harm caused to the patients' trust in the profession will almost certainly bleed over into their trust in individual members of it. They will have little reason to trust them if they don't trust their profession.

In short, conscientious refusals can damage patient trust—in objectors, their profession, and fellow professionals—by undercutting the reliance patients have in the competence of objectors. This outcome is certainly harmful, but notice that it is not inevitable; for conscientious refusals need not reveal to patients that objectors lack competence, of a non-moral or moral variety. The objectors may not claim to be technically incompetent or say anything that indicates a lack of such competence, or even do anything that signals a deficiency in moral competence. The objectors may show enough sympathy for their patients that the patients do not lose confidence in their ability to be morally responsible. Indeed, the patients might believe that the objectors have this ability but are simply not using it when they conscientiously refuse to provide abortion services; in other words, they are not acting responsibly despite being capable of doing so. Patients could very well have this attitude toward objectors, although it does not target the objectors' competence. Instead, it aims at something like their goodwill.

1.2 Reliance on Goodwill

Normally, trust requires reliance not simply on the competence of trustees, but also on their commitment (or motivation) to do what one trusts them to

---

[15] Here, the patient could be questioning the competence of those who run the profession to do their job properly or alternatively the goodwill of these people toward the population that the profession serves. Unlike with patient trust in objectors, I will not, in the interests of space, deconstruct patient trust in professions or its members when discussing the effects of conscientious refusal on this trust.

do (McLeod 2015). Baier argues that this commitment stems from goodwill (see also Jones 1996). She uses the criterion of reliance on goodwill to explain why one would assume that trustees are motivated to do what one trusts them to do, but also to distinguish trust from mere reliance:

> What is the difference between trusting others and mere relying on them? It seems to be reliance on their good will toward one, as distinct from their dependable habits, or only on their dependably exhibited fear, anger, or other motives compatible with ill will toward one, or on motives not directed toward one at all.   (Baier 1986, 234)

Here, goodwill should be understood as care or concern for the other, which itself could be grounded in fellow feeling, benevolence, conscientiousness, or the like (Jones 1996, 7). In trusting people, we rely on their goodwill, so understood. Although some philosophers object to this theory,[16] I believe that it (or something close to it)[17] captures well the trust that many people have in health care professionals. They trust them because they feel that they will show care or concern for them, whether out of duty and conscientiousness, pure benevolence, or fellow feeling. People have a sense that they *can* rely on health care professionals in this way, moreover, because of a climate in which these professionals are expected to care for others (those who have significant health care needs) and to recognize as their primary duty the need to care for their patients.

Conscientious refusals can certainly damage the reliance that patients have on the goodwill of their health care professionals. For example, patients who trust their physician enough to request abortion services but are refused

---

[16] For example, Richard Holton suggests that reliance on goodwill is absent in certain trust relationships including relationships between con artists and their marks (1994). Since I am not claiming that reliance on goodwill is necessary for trust (see note 7), however, this concern does not apply to my theory. One criticism that does relate to it, granted, comes from Jones. She worries about interpreting "goodwill" as I have here (and as she does in her earlier work; 1996)—so that it encompasses "benevolence, honesty, conscientiousness, integrity, and the like"—because it is then "a meaningless catchall that merely reports the presence of some positive motive, and one that may or may not even be directed toward the truster" (2012, 67). I am afraid I don't see, however, how interpreting the term so broadly makes it meaningless. Rather, doing so is useful because it allows us to capture the many different positive motives people can have for honoring the trust that is placed in them (see Walker 2006).

[17] Perhaps, we feel the people we trust *ought to* show goodwill toward us, not simply that they *will* do so. In other words, we have a normative expectation of their goodwill. This is Zac Cogley's theory (2012), which he says solves the problem of the con artist, as described in note 16. Although I find this view promising, I don't support it here because Baier's view is more generally accepted and I don't think it matters for my purposes who's correct: Baier or Cogley.

them on grounds of conscience could easily question whether their physician feels goodwill toward them. Patients who ask for an abortion are usually in a vulnerable position (as are patients who request similar services, such as EC; see Chapter 2). They need the abortion so that they can protect their education, children's well-being, financial security, health, or the like (Finer et al. 2005; see also Chapter 2). Usually, patients decide on an abortion for such reasons, *not*—as some anti-abortion people would have it—because they are selfish or view abortion as a form of birth control, or because people close to them have pressured them to have an abortion.[18] Given the circumstances that lead many patients to choose abortion, it is understandable that some who are refused abortion services by a conscientious objector would feel that the objector lacks care or concern for them. The reaction would probably be, "How could my well-being matter so little to this person that they would not try to help me?" The response will be even stronger, of course, in cases where the objector is the only health care professional around who is available to assist the patient.

The above sort of reaction to a conscientious refusal could also be explained by the climate of trust, insofar as it concerns the moral character of people who have abortions. Patients could easily believe that their well-being matters very little to objectors, because they (the patients) view the objection through the lens of abortion stigma (i.e., stigma surrounding an abortion; see Cockrill and Nack 2013, Cockrill et al. 2013, and Kumar et al. 2009). For instance, they may know that the social perception of women who have abortions is that they are irresponsible, selfish, or the like (a perception that is more or less strong depending on prevailing social views about abortions). When their physician conscientiously refuses to offer them abortion services, they will then assume that their physician has this perception of them—that is, if they present as women. Consequently, they will feel they can no longer trust in the physician's goodwill. The same effect could occur with refusals to dispense EC, because, as discussed in Chapter 2, there is stigma surrounding patients' use of EC that is similar to abortion stigma.

Conscientious refusals and the social climate that surrounds them can therefore destroy or disrupt the reliance patients have on the goodwill of objectors. They are likely to affect the patients' reliance on their goodwill

[18] See, e.g., Pro-Life America's "Testimonials of Women Who Have Had Abortions" at http://www.prolife.com/ABRTWM2.html, or the Pennsylvania Pro-Life Federation statement on "Why Women Have Abortions" at http://www.paprolife.org/why-women-have-abortions/ (retrieved May 20, 2019).

insofar as it extends not only to abortion care, but also to other forms of care. Patients who ask, "How could my well-being matter so little to this person that they would deny me an abortion?" or who think the objector views them with moral suspicion will, no doubt, be reluctant to depend on their goodwill in other contexts.

Patients who feel that they can no longer rely on the goodwill of objecting health care professionals will also be inclined to question the trustworthiness of the profession itself if it permits conscientious objections. Normally, physicians are allowed by their professional associations to conscientiously refuse to perform abortions (though often only if they give a referral to a health care professional who is willing and able to do the abortion; Chavkin et al. 2013, S50; IWHC 2017). Patients who investigate whether a conscientious objection that they experience is permissible, and who find out that it is according to the objector's professional organization, could certainly lose trust in that organization and residually in other members of it. They will have discovered that the trust they had was misplaced.

Damage to trust from an inability to rely on objectors' goodwill can therefore be far-reaching. Conscientious objections can harm patients greatly by interfering with their trust in this way. To be clear, these actions need not have this effect, however; patients can assume that physicians who conscientiously refuse their requests for abortion services still feel goodwill toward them. The physicians might give them a proper referral for an abortion, for example, which in turn allows them to continue to rely on their physician's goodwill. The physicians might also state their refusal in such a respectful and compassionate way—a way that deflects any stigma the patients might experience—that the patients are not left questioning their goodwill. Alternatively, the patients might believe they can still depend on their physician's goodwill even if the physician is *not* very respectful or compassionate toward them. The reason is that the patients feel guilty or ashamed about asking for an abortion in the first place (as some patients do),[19] and they therefore don't blame their physician for denying their request and even assume that the physician shows moral concern for them in doing so.

To sum up what I believe I've established so far: conscientious refusals can, though need not, disrupt patients' reliance on the goodwill or competence of

---

[19] See, e.g., Cockrill and Nack (2013, 980), Kumar et al. (2009), and Norris et al. (2011). These authors interpret such feelings as "manifestations of internalized abortion stigma" (Kumar et al. 2009, 633).

objectors. They needn't do either, in fact. Patients who are refused abortion services by respectful and compassionate objectors could still rely on their goodwill and their competence. Nonetheless, the patients' trust in the physicians would be damaged, for they wouldn't trust them any longer to provide them, at the very least, with abortion services. Now what feature of trust can explain this fact?

1.3 Expectation about Some Shared Values

Usually, in trusting people, we expect them to share enough of (or enough of a commitment to) our values that we can indeed trust them.[20] This element of trust can help to explain our optimism that the people we trust will be motivated to do what we trust them to do. There must be more to this optimism than mere reliance on goodwill, that is, if we can rely on people's goodwill without trusting them, which is the case with the patients who encounter the compassionate and caring conscientious objector. They no longer trust them to provide abortion services, simply because they can no longer expect them to value these services enough to offer them.

People can, and often do, have expectations about sharing some values with health care professionals. Prior experience with these professionals can help to explain this fact, but so can social climate, which is infused with norms about what health care professionals are committed to doing, and about what patients are entitled to receive in terms of their health care. The professions themselves shape this climate—for example, using codes of ethics for their members, often proudly displayed in members' offices—and so do bodies such as government, licensing boards, and insurance companies. In the case of abortion access in Canada, for instance, provincial and territorial governments deem abortion to be a medically necessary service and fund most abortions on these grounds. Moreover, the only health care professionals licensed to perform surgical abortions or prescribe the abortion pill are physicians.[21] Although physicians are free, outside of emergency situations, to conscientiously object to provide abortion services themselves, usually

---

[20] These people need not share our values in the sense that they reflectively endorse them. They need only be committed to them, where the commitment could arise ultimately out of self-interest (e.g., an interest in avoiding a charge of professional misconduct).

[21] On policy with respect to the abortion pill Mifepristone (which goes under the name Mifegymiso in Canada), see https://www.cpso.on.ca/Physicians/Policies-Guidance/Statements-Positions/Mifegymiso (retrieved May 16, 2019).

they must give proper referrals for them. Anyone in Canada with even partial knowledge of these facts surrounding abortion access could easily expect a physician to be committed to providing abortion services, or at least referrals for abortion, and consequently trust a physician to do so.

Conscientious refusals can damage patients' trust, however, by undermining their expectation about shared values. Patients who trust their physician to provide them with a referral for an abortion must expect the physician to value doing so.[22] In the event that the physician refuses to offer this service, the patients' expectation will be disappointed.[23] Their trust will be damaged, if only because of this fact.

More needs to be said in favor of the view that patient trust often involves an expectation about shared values,[24] particularly if the expectation amounts to the thought that the physician *will* do specific things for the patient, such as provide a referral for an abortion. Some might question whether such an attitude is compatible with patients giving health care professionals discretionary power over their interests (i.e., power to use their discretion when acting in their interests). Granting such authority to the trustee is an important element of trust, according to many theories of it, especially Baier's.[25] What is more, discretionary power is a defining feature of fiduciary relationships, which is the sort of relationship that physicians have (and other health care professionals can have) with their patients, as I argue in Chapter 5. Would an expectation about shared values, especially values in favor of respecting patient autonomy surrounding abortion, not seriously limit the discretionary power that patients confer on physicians, and in turn, limit the trust that they place in them? If patients expect that in the

[22] Granted, in some climates—for example, where abortion stigma is high and there are clear norms in favor of physicians' right to conscience with respect to abortion—patients may ask for abortions merely in the *hope* that their physician will accede to their request, not with an expectation that they will do so. But then the patients simply have hope, not trust.

[23] Notice that in many cases of conscientious refusal, the expectation about having some shared values will be undermined along with the reliance on goodwill; the patients will be surprised that their physician is not committed to the relevant service and will assume, because of this fact, that the physician is not sufficiently concerned about their welfare.

[24] According to Jones, such an expectation is not necessary for trust (2012, 77–8). I agree. My claim is only that this expectation is a feature within our cluster concept of trust. See note 7.

[25] Baier argues that trust involves entrusting people with discretionary power to care for things that we care about. In her view, this power helps to explain the special vulnerability that we incur in trusting people (1986, 239); they may use their discretionary power in poor or arbitrary ways and therefore cause us harm. Interestingly, a legitimate expectation about shared values—an expectation informed, for instance, by accepted norms of a profession—can help to determine what should count as a poor or arbitrary use of discretionary power. Professionals who use their discretionary power in ways that betray a lack of commitment to these norms would be using their power poorly or arbitrarily.

end, physicians will simply provide them with certain services—those that they want for themselves—then they do not trust in their physicians' discretionary power to decide which services they should receive.

To respond to this concern, I agree that an expectation about some shared values restricts the amount of discretionary power that the truster gives to the trustee; however, this power often needs to be reined in and does not have to be complete for trust to occur. Consider it would be foolish for most patients to trust health care professionals without *any* expectation about what they value, thereby giving them *absolute* discretionary power. Moreover, patients who expect physicians to value certain services, along with patients' choices in favor of these services, could still rely on physicians' discretion: about, say in abortion cases, the best way to inform patients about abortion, which method of abortion (surgical or medical) is right for them, or whether they have properly consented to an abortion. Patient trust can, and indeed normally should, therefore involve an expectation about some shared values.

I hope to have said enough about this expectation to show that it is normally a feature of patient trust and that conscientious refusals can weaken or destroy it.[26] Consider now what affect this result can have on patient trust in the profession and in its members more generally. If patients discover that the profession is fine with its members not being committed to certain values of the profession in their practice—values that the patients themselves hold—then they will likely question the profession's own commitment to them (e.g., to abortion access). And as a result, their trust in the profession will decrease, as will their trust in its members generally. They will no longer be able to assume that these people cherish the relevant values, because their profession does not do so.

Thus, a final way in which trust can be lost because of conscientious refusals is that they challenge patients' expectation of there being some shared values between them and the objecting professional, or them and the profession and its members. As we have seen, these denials of service can also damage the reliance patients have on the goodwill or competence of the trustee. Since conscientious refusals can undermine patient trust in any or all of these ways, patient trust must be at stake in allowing these refusals to occur. It is a likely casualty of permissive policies toward conscientious objection.

I do want to acknowledge that some conscientious refusals could be trust-enhancing, because of how they occur.[27] For instance, health care professionals

---

[26]   For more on this aspect of trust, see McLeod (2002), especially chapter 2, pp. 27–31.
[27]   Thanks to an anonymous referee from OUP for alerting me to this objection.

who make a conscientious objection without revealing a lack of competence and goodwill could be trusted *more* by their patients as a result, not to provide the service that morally offends them to be sure, but to provide other health care services. The reason for this heightened trust would be the openness and honesty that the objectors display about their values. Similarly, conscientious refusals that are accompanied by proper referrals, where the patients understand that the profession has a policy in favor of such referrals, could increase the trust the patients have in both the objector and the relevant profession, specifically because of the concern that a proper referral demonstrates for patient well-being. I agree such an outcome is possible, and I want to emphasize that my conclusion is only that conscientious refusals are *likely* to damage patient trust. At the same time, I believe my argument shows that the potential these refusals have to decrease patient trust is greater than their potential to do otherwise. The reason why is that to influence trust negatively, a refusal simply has to undermine *one* of the features of trust I have discussed (assuming that each feature plays a key role in trust relationships in health care), and there is more than one way that damage can occur to each of these features.

In response to my position on trust and conscientious refusals, one might ask whether it's possible to regulate these refusals so that the threat they pose to patient trust is seriously reduced or eliminated but they themselves are not prohibited. Better yet, perhaps one could regulate them in a way that would enhance patient trust, say by matching objecting professionals with patients who share many of their values. These considerations are relevant to Section 2, where I discuss a policy recommended in the bioethics literature for promoting the trust of patients *and* the freedom of conscience of health care professionals, more specifically of physicians.

2.   Responding to the Damage: Through Morals Matching?

Most bioethicists do not seem to notice the damage that conscientious refusals can do to patient trust. An exception is Lynch. As a strategy for trying to minimize—even eliminate—this damage, she proposes what she calls "Morals Matching," which is part of her institutional compromise to conflicts of conscience in medicine. Let me describe Lynch's proposal, and then argue that as a method for promoting patient trust, Morals Matching should be rejected.

Lynch claims that the best way to approach the problem of conscientious refusals is to adopt an institutional solution in which licensing boards help patients match themselves with physicians who have similar moral values. In her view, individual physicians are not professionally obligated to ensure that patients have access to services, and therefore need not refrain from exercising freedom of conscience in their practice (2008, 41). Instead, the profession as a whole has this responsibility. (*It* is the gatekeeper to these services; it has a legal monopoly over them (71).) Moreover, it should fulfill this responsibility by having licensing boards encourage Morals Matching. Lynch develops this framework for the sake not of patient trust, but of other values such as the freedom of conscience of physicians. Nevertheless, she claims that an "added benefit" of Morals Matching is that it would improve trust in patient–physician relationships (90), a view that clearly trades on the importance for trust of an expectation about some shared values. I will explain how Lynch's system of Morals Matching is supposed to work in practice, and then evaluate it using examples involving, again, conscientious refusals by physicians to provide abortions.

According to Lynch, licensing boards should require that physicians register their conscientious objections with them, and then should make the registry available to patients so they can match themselves with physicians who are willing to provide the services they seek (and perhaps even refuse to offer services they, the patients, find morally offensive).[28] In addition, the boards would be obligated to ensure there are enough willing physicians—in particular, physicians prepared to perform controversial procedures, such as abortions—in different geographical areas. Last, they would need to encourage patients to "check the registry of unwilling physicians before seeking care and to select only those doctors who match their own preferences" (217). Such a system, although designed by Lynch with physicians in mind, could certainly work for other health care professionals who could be matched with patients by licensing boards.

Lynch recognizes that not all patients would consult or be able to consult the registry that she proposes. Not all of them would be aware of it. What is more, using it "may not be an option in an emergency and may be too much to expect of the young or vulnerable patient" (217). Consequently,

---

[28] Lynch refers to different versions of Moral Matching: what we can call "Weak Morals Matching" and "Strong Morals Matching." With the former, patients are able to find physicians who will perform the services they seek, while with the latter, they are also able to choose physicians who will "deny undesirable services to others" (93). According to Lynch, weak matches are more important than strong ones. She therefore obligates licensing boards to ensure there are enough *willing* physicians available, but not that there are enough *unwilling* physicians: in other words, to facilitate weak matches, not strong ones.

Lynch lays out certain duties—what she calls "nonnegotiable" or "collective" duties—which all physicians share, and which unwilling physicians must fulfill when patients who are unaware of their conscientious objections come to them for health care.

Lynch's list of nonnegotiable duties includes notifying patients promptly of one's moral refusals, informing them of all of their treatment options, and providing care in emergencies (215).[29] Notably, the list *excludes* providing a proper referral.[30] Lynch insists that unwilling physicians should not be obligated to accept patients if after disclosing their moral beliefs to them, they discover that they and the patient make a bad morals match. They also should never be required, outside of an emergency, to offer services they find morally offensive, or to refer patients for these services to willing physicians.[31] Lynch suggests that conscientious objectors must provide emergency care if they are competent to do so; however, she does not prohibit them from being *deliberately incompetent* because they conscientiously refused to be trained in the relevant services.

Beyond fulfilling their nonnegotiable duties, Lynch believes that physicians should be able to conduct their practice in a way that fits with their moral or religious values. The result would most likely be ethical "subspecializations," in which some, perhaps many, physicians have their own distinct set of professional ethical obligations (2008, 88).[32] Lynch refers favorably to there being many ethical "subroles" for physicians, even "as many strains of medicine as there are value systems" (87).

Let me comment on the possible benefits of Morals Matching, focusing again on elements that concern patient trust, before turning to the moral hazards of such a system (which may seem obvious at this point). Patients who use the registry of unwilling physicians to avoid encountering physicians of this sort should not experience conscientious refusals and any resulting damage to their trust. As well, the trust that patients have in the physicians they choose may be deeper than it otherwise would be, because of the

[29] She also adds to the list of nonnegotiable duties a duty to avoid religious proselytism and "moral arrogance" (215).

[30] In lieu of having a requirement that objectors refer patients to willing physicians, Lynch says that unwilling physicians *could* (though may not) be obligated to encourage patients to consult their licensing board for information on how to access services (236).

[31] Lynch justifies these elements of her view, in part, by saying that being refused care is merely inconvenient for patients who could simply go to another physician. On why this line of reasoning is unpersuasive, see Chapter 2.

[32] As Lynch says, physicians are able to choose medical subspecializations, such as being a pediatrician who focuses exclusively on children with gender dysphoria, so why not ethical subspecializations (88)?

"deep-value pairings" that Morals Matching permits and indeed encourages (Lynch 2008, 92). Patients—some of them at least—will be able to match themselves with physicians whose moral values closely align with their own. They will be able to do that because of the registry, which will allow patients either to avoid or seek out physicians who are unwilling to offer certain services (i.e., depending on whether the patients value or object to these services). A further source of deep-value pairings will be clinics that have particular religious, ethical, or political orientations. Lynch suggests that Morals Matching would promote the creation of centers of this kind, which seems right given the emphasis on ethical subspecializations. She gives examples of Christian clinics (socially conservative ones), including the Tepeyac Family Center in Fairfax, VA (now Tepeyac OB/GYN),[33] which strives to combine "the best of modern medicine with the healing presence of Jesus Christ" (quoted in Lynch 2008, 96). But one could also give non-Christian, non-conservative examples, such as the Feminist Women's Health Center in Atlanta, GA, which aims "to provide…gynecological healthcare to all who need it without judgment" and to "advance reproductive health, rights and justice."[34] If—as Lynch says—trust is "enhanced through alliance on moral issues" (90), then clinics like these should allow for deep trust relationships between health care professionals and patients.

For many patients who seek an abortion and feel entitled to get one, the opportunity to receive care from a professional whose moral values match their own with respect to abortion is surely ideal. The trust they would have in the professional who provides them with an abortion would be great. Thus, if Morals Matching led to the creation of more clinics like the Feminist Women's Health Center—those that endeavor to provide non-judgmental compassionate abortion care—then such a system must be beneficial from the perspective of these patients.

To conclude, however, that Morals Matching is itself ideal because it would foster high levels of trust would be too quick. For it would not necessarily have this effect, and what is more, it would pose significant barriers to trust. Consider that such a system would not guarantee the creation of clinics like the Feminist Women's Health Center, and thus could not promise the deep trust relationships that could occur at these clinics. Recall that with Morals Matching, licensing boards must ensure there are enough willing physicians available. But they needn't confirm there are enough willing

[33] See http://tepeyacobgyn.com (retrieved May 20, 2019).
[34] See http://www.feministcenter.org (retrieved May 20, 2019).

physicians who have certain political or moral beliefs. In some socio-political environments—for example, those where anti-abortion sentiment is widespread and entrenched—the boards will likely have to give serious incentives for physicians to provide services like abortions. And if that were the case, then many of the "willing" physicians that the boards identify would not have the moral values that patients would want them to have. As a result, Morals Matching would not produce the "deep-value pairings" that Lynch predicts, and would not improve, as she puts it, "the level of trust that is so integral to successful medical encounters" (90).

Even where Morals Matching was successful in creating deep-value pairings, it could not always sustain them because the relevant parties may change their values. Physicians who notified patients ahead of time about their ethical subspecialty could change it partway through their relationships with patients, which is not something Lynch opposes.[35] The patients too could change their values. Lynch admits that some patients who were "previously prepared to accept limitations on the services that [their] physician is willing to provide may change [their] mind down the road" (217). Included among these patients will very likely be some who want an abortion. Evidence suggests that the incidence of abortions among people who identify, or once identified, as pro-life and anti-abortion is quite high.[36] Patients with these values might flock to clinics like the Tepeyac Family Center when they are available. But then if they find themselves in an unwanted pregnancy and actually want an abortion, they will no longer be able to trust their physician. Their lack of trust would stem from a change in their values—presumably, they would no longer believe that abortion is *strictly* prohibited—or simply from an inability to rely on the goodwill or competence of their physician (i.e., in relation to their need for an abortion).

One might argue that a system of Morals Matching shouldn't have to accommodate cases like the ones just described, where patients are anti-abortion but then request an abortion. The reason is that the patients' set of values is simply incoherent.[37] Although the same sort of objection could

---

[35] Indeed, she suggests that physicians should have the freedom to change their moral values without penalty. More specifically, she comments that physicians who develop new ethical objections to services whilst in relationships with patients should simply notify them of this fact so that they have the opportunity to find a new physician (218).

[36] Despite there being strong anti-abortion views among evangelical Christians and Catholics generally, "one in five abortion patients [in the United States] identify themselves as evangelical…Christian, and Catholic women have abortions at a rate similar to that of all women" (Cockrill et al. 2013, 86). To read about the experience of one woman who was anti-abortion but then had an abortion, see Anonymous/xojane (2015).

[37] This objection comes from an anonymous reviewer from OUP.

be made, of course, about physicians who change their values, let me focus on this objection concerning patients. I have three responses to offer. First, because the patients may have revised their values in response to experiential knowledge they have gained while being in an unwanted pregnancy, their values may not be incoherent at all. Second, even if their values were somewhat incoherent, the patients might still deserve or need to receive the services they are requesting and to receive them, moreover, from a physician with whom they are in an existing relationship. In that case, a system of Morals Matching would have to accommodate them. Third, and most importantly for my purposes, regardless of whether the patients' values are incoherent, I'm assuming that because of how their values have shifted, they can no longer trust their physician, which speaks against Lynch's claim that Morals Matching would enhance trust between patients and physicians.

In summary, Morals Matching would not allow all patients to have high levels of trust in their physicians or even to maintain trust in them. But let me turn to what I take to be a graver problem, which is that this system would seriously limit the trust that patients can have in any physician qua physician (i.e., in their social role as a physician). I contend that this, along with other effects of Morals Matching, would also seriously jeopardize the trust that patients have in the medical profession. The same problem would occur, moreover, if Morals Matching were introduced in other health care professions, such as pharmacy.

The ability to trust physicians qua physicians is a worry in particular for patients who do not consult, or are not able to consult, the registry of unwilling physicians. As Lynch suggests, these are often the most vulnerable patients. (They are very young, very old, or very poor; they are facing a health care emergency; etc.). Without using the registry, patients would not know what a physician they approach stands for, beyond fulfilling the non-negotiable duties that Lynch lists. They would not be able to rely on the physician to show substantial care or concern for them: that is, to have the level of goodwill that would motivate them to put their health in the physician's hands. Perhaps they could do so in an emergency, because of the nonnegotiable duty to treat in an emergency. But notice that with Morals Matching, the ability to trust a physician in an emergency would not be guaranteed either, for some physicians will be deliberately incompetent (e.g., to perform abortions) because of a conscientious objection. Lynch simply accepts this outcome and says, "it is sufficient to limit emergency obligations to those already competent to provide the service the patient seeks," even though, as she adds, "[t]his may leave some patients without a physician in a true emergency" (228). The effect of such an arrangement on patient trust would surely be very negative, however.[38] Patients would not be justified in trusting all, or even *any*, emergency room doctors to provide them with morally controversial services, since any of them could be conscientious objectors.

A further possibility with Morals Matching is that emergency room physicians do not construe, and are not obligated to construe, a patient's situation as an emergency, even though many of us would do so. (For a discussion about the nature of emergencies and also how objecting health care professionals can view emergencies differently than patients, see Chapter 2.) These physicians could be competent to do what the patient needs them to do, but nevertheless could not be trusted to do it, because they would not feel or *be* duty-bound to offer the relevant care. While discussing what characterizes an emergency, Lynch gives the real-life example of a patient whose water broke in the second trimester of a pregnancy and who would likely miscarry within weeks (227). Not having an abortion right away would put the patient at significant risk of an infection that could ultimately cause infertility or even death.[39] Despite the severity of these circumstances, Lynch views the case as "marginal" and leaves room for physicians, licensing boards, and others (e.g., hospitals) to deem it a "non-emergency." If indeed such an outcome is possible with Morals Matching, then this system *must* constrain the degree to which patients can trust physicians qua physicians in emergencies.

In my view, the most serious problem with Morals Matching is that it threatens our ability to trust physicians qua physicians. This problem exists, moreover, because under this system, being a physician—that is, occupying the role of physician—would not signal that one is trustworthy in ways that many of us think physicians should be trustworthy. We tend to believe, for example, that physicians should be committed to putting patient needs above their personal interests. Indeed, inhabiting the role of physician is usually a "standing social signal" that one has this commitment (Jones 2012, 76).[40] One indicates that one can be trusted to honor such an obligation by

---

[38] That is assuming the details of Morals Matching become widely known, which is something Lynch intends to have happen (218).

[39] The patient is Kathleen Hutchins and her local hospital would not allow her to have the abortion until she developed an infection (Lynch 227, citing Erdely 2007). Her physician, Dr. Goldner, reportedly drove her 80 miles to the nearest hospital where she could have an abortion (Rowland 2004, 290–1).

[40] Karen Jones argues that people who are truly (or "richly") trustworthy signal their trustworthiness to others and can be aided in doing so by standing social signals of their trustworthiness (2012).

presenting oneself as a physician (e.g., by wearing the white coat, displaying a medical diploma on one's wall, etc.).

Morals Matching would disrupt standing social signals of the trustworthiness of physicians for the reasons I've articulated. (And clearly, it would do the same for other health care professionals.) It would alter the climate of trust so that people could no longer make what are now common presumptions about the trustworthy of physicians. As a result, people would find it difficult to approach physicians who are unknown to them about their health care needs, simply because they wouldn't know whether or how much they can trust them. Perhaps the physicians occupy an ethical subrole that they, the patients, find morally problematic and that would not allow the physicians to adequately serve their health care needs.[41] This possibility would garner distrust or at least inhibit trust among patients who do not use Lynch's registry of unwilling physicians.

In addition to compromising patients' trust in physicians qua physicians, Morals Matching would also likely diminish the public's trust in the medical profession. The first problem would lead to the second, in fact, because if people cannot trust physicians qua physicians, then they are not likely to trust their profession. It is doubtful that under Morals Matching, the profession would be trustworthy regardless, because it could not ensure, even in emergencies, access to services that it deems essential. It could not demand that all physicians know how to perform these services (those that are part of their specialty) and it would not require referrals for them. How does that square with the services being *essential*? Sensible patients would ask this question, and would in turn doubt the trustworthiness of the profession.

In short, although Morals Matching could be beneficial in terms of allowing some patients (those who do not modify their values!) to have deep trust relationships with physicians, it would also be harmful because it would inhibit trust in physicians qua physicians and in the profession of medicine. It would have this impact, in particular, on the most vulnerable patients. The focus of this discussion has been on physicians, although there is no reason to think that a system of Morals Matching would go any better for pharmacists or other health care professionals. Given these drawbacks, which are very serious, we should not settle for this system as our chosen method

---

[41] Lynch suggests that with her model, patients should be able to presume that physicians "are operating on some core, consensus morality unless they inform patients to the contrary" (89; quoting Veatch 1991, 153). But why would patients assume this and approach a professional who is new to them with a trusting attitude given what is normally at stake for them in trusting a physician? Lynch does not tell us why.

of preventing the damage to patient trust that conscientious refusals can cause. Rather, we should seek out a different method. We should pursue, more specifically, a strategy that would permit us to have reasonably clear expectations about what health care professionals stand for as professionals, which, as we have seen, is important for patient trust. The prioritizing approach to conscientious refusals that I defend in Chapters 5 and 6 allows for such expectations. It does so because it requires individual professionals to ensure that patients who request standard services that are medically indicated for them receive these services, either from the professionals themselves or from a trustworthy colleague.

3. Conclusion

My aim in this chapter has been to show that conscientious refusals can seriously jeopardize the trust patients have in health care professionals and professions. This conduct can destroy or diminish different elements of patient trust, including reliance on goodwill and competence, and an expectation about some shared values. Its effect on trust also reveals that the last of these features is among the cluster of features that make up our concept of trust and is key to our trust in health care professionals. Indicating the same thing is Lynch's Morals Matching, which makes sense as a solution to the problem of trust and conscientious refusals only if an expectation about some shared values is a crucial part of trust relations in health care. I have raised grave doubts about whether Morals Matching is the best way to encourage this expectation, however, along with the other dimensions of patient trust. Undeniably, in my opinion, if we care about the trust of patients, especially very vulnerable ones, then we should fervidly oppose Morals Matching.

PART II

REGULATING CONSCIENTIOUS REFUSALS

4

Why Not Compromise?

Based on Chapters 1 to 3, we can assume that serious interests often *are* at
stake for the main parties to conflicts of conscience in reproductive health
care. We can say that what lies in the balance for many conscientious objectors is their moral integrity, which is a common claim in bioethics, although
in Chapter 1, I interpreted "moral integrity" differently than most bioethicists do (i.e., in terms not of moral unity or protecting one's identity, but of
acting in accordance with one's best moral judgment).[1] On the other hand,
for many patients, the interests at stake include their freedom not from
mere inconvenience—as some bioethicists would have it—but from harm
in the form of a loss of reproductive autonomy, moral identity, a sense of
security, or the ability to trust in health care professionals and professions.
That is true, I argued in Chapters 2 and 3, for typical cases of conscientious
refusal in reproductive health care, particularly those involving abortion
and emergency contraception, although it stands to reason that some of the
harms I identified there—including the damage to patient trust—would
occur in other cases of conscientious refusal as well.

Given that with typical refusals (at least), there are usually important
interests at stake on both sides, one might suppose that the best solution in
terms of health policy is to strike a compromise. The goal there would be to
find some sort of middle-ground solution, one that would protect both sets
of interests to some degree. Many bioethicists take this sort of approach—
what Wicclair aptly names "the compromise approach"—to regulating conflicts of conscience in health care (2011). In other words, they argue for a
general policy on conscientious refusals (a policy for all types of refusal) that
amounts to a compromise. These authors include Wicclair (2011), Benjamin
(1990), Blustein (1993), Lynch (2008), and Dan Brock (2008), among others.
Despite its popularity, I will argue that the compromise approach will not
work, not for many if not most typical refusals in reproductive health care.

---

[1] As I mentioned in Chapter 1, in moving forward, it is important that one accepts not my
account of moral integrity and conscience, but that usually something as valuable as moral
integrity is at stake in denying conscientious objectors protection for their conscience.

Conscience in Reproductive Health Care: Prioritizing Patient Interests. Carolyn McLeod, Oxford University Press (2020).
© Carolyn McLeod.
DOI: 10.1093/oso/9780198732723.001.0001

The problem is that the prospects of reaching a compromise in these cases—one that all parties could reasonably accept—are dim.[2] I conclude therefore that we should reject the compromise approach to developing any policy specific to typical conscientious refusals, and that since these refusals are common among and paradigmatic of conscientious refusals in health care, we should reject any general policy that aims at compromise as well.

There are two main sections to this chapter. Section 1 looks at the nature of compromises and considers what makes a compromise true (i.e., genuine) as well as good. There can be true compromises that are not good compromises, and any theory about compromises should be able to explain the difference. There are probably multiple ways to understand this difference and there appears to be no canonical way to do so in the literature on compromises, and so I stipulate that for a compromise to be true (or genuine) there must be reasons for it, and for a compromise to be good there must be good reasons for it. The details about true and good (as well as false and bad) compromises are important when discussing conscientious refusals in health care, yet they are mostly missing from the bioethical literature on this topic. Those who defend the compromise approach tend to ignore these details,[3] but they do so at their peril, in my opinion. Thus, I spend considerable time in Section 1 examining the nature of compromises.

In Section 2, I argue that it is very difficult, if not impossible, to formulate a policy on conscientious refusals that would constitute a true and good compromise for most objectors, again typical ones in reproductive health care (i.e., those who disapprove of reproductive practices that threaten "unborn lives"). Of course, it matters as well whether there could be a good compromise for patients, although advocates of the compromise approach ("*compromise theorists*" for short) usually do not discuss this matter. For my purposes, it is enough to show that the compromise approach will not work for one of the main parties to these conflicts. I have chosen to focus on objectors, rather than patients, because I want to counter claims by compromise theorists that their strategy will work for most objectors. I also want to bring in the viewpoints of typical objectors, which, to this point, are mostly missing from this book. (I actually get the language of "true" as

---

[2] Even if the prospects were better, it is questionable whether the compromise approach is appropriate given that it treats the objector's interests as though they were on a par with patient interests or interests of the public in access to care. The latter sets of interests may have to take priority for reasons that concern the objector's duties as a health care professional. I discuss this possibility in Chapters 5 and 6.

[3] Benjamin (1990) is an exception.

opposed to "false" compromises from them, along with the idea that false compromises are those they have no reason to make.)[4] Their perspectives, together with facts about the nature of compromise and about conscientious refusals, support the conclusion that a good compromise is not a live option for many (if again not most) conscientious objectors.

Section 2 critically assesses the policy solution that compromise theorists recommend most often, which is to allow conscientious objectors—in many though not all circumstances[5]—to refuse to perform the service they object to so long as they provide a proper referral for it, which is a referral "to another professional willing and able to provide the service" (Brock 2008, 194). This solution forms part of what Dan Brock calls the "conventional compromise," which also requires that objectors inform patients of their health care options and not "impose an unreasonable burden" on them (2008, 194). Since the part of this proposal that has generated the most controversy is the referral requirement, I will concentrate on it and for simplicity, will allow the term "conventional compromise" to refer mainly to it. I will use this compromise to illustrate the problems I see with the compromise approach, although my concerns with it extend to other sorts of compromises proposed by bioethicists for conflicts of conscience in health care. (An example is the "institutional compromise" developed by Lynch (2008) and discussed in Chapter 3.)

The upshot of this chapter is that policy requirements like giving proper referrals cannot be grounded in compromise. At the same time, requirements of this sort are important for guaranteeing that patients have access to standard services. While compromise theorists tend to agree with this last point, they do not provide the justification needed to support policies that would ensure access. We need a different strategy for regulating conscientious refusals if patient access is important to us. I argue in Chapters 5 and 6 that the approach we need is one that prioritizes patient interests and the interests of the public in public health and equitable access to care.

1. Varieties of Compromise

Let me begin by discussing the nature of compromise, and by introducing an example that has nothing to do with conscientious refusals in health care

---

[4] See, e.g., Polizogopoulos (2014, 21), and also http://www.consciencelaws.org/ethics/ethics012.aspx (retrieved May 21, 2019).
[5] Emergency situations are an exception, for example.

but which should help us to better understand compromises. The example comes from Daniel Stoljar and concerns the creation of the city he lives in, Canberra:

> The story of Canberra, the capital of Australia, is roughly as follows. In 1901, when what is called 'Federation' occurred—that is, when the six colonies then occupying the territory of Australia decided to join forces and become one colony—it was naturally felt that there should be a capital city. But the rulers of the two most powerful cities, Sydney and Melbourne, could not agree which of them it was to be. (Nobody took seriously the claims of any other city.) So it was decided to build a completely new city more or less midway between them. In short, Canberra is constitutively connected to compromise.   (Stoljar 2009, 113; see also Davison et al. 2003)[6]

I'll use this case to illustrate the distinctions between true and false, and good and bad compromises. I'll also introduce another distinction: between standard and non-standard compromises. Non-standard compromises are particularly relevant to conscientious refusals because the conventional compromise—again, that health care professionals can object so long as they give a proper referral—falls into this category. (What is conventional about this solution is that it is commonly used to settle conflicts of conscience in health care. It is not conventional *as a* compromise; it does not count, in other words, as a standard compromise. In an effort to make this clear, I will put "conventional" in quotation marks when referring to the "conventional" compromise.) The fact that the "conventional" compromise is non-standard is significant, although it is largely absent from bioethical discussions about compromise and conscientious refusals. This compromise is also meant to be true and good, but it's probably neither when the refusals at issue are typical ones in reproductive health care.

1.1 Standard Compromises

The core features of standard compromises appear in the Canberra case and are highlighted in philosophical work on compromise. Let me list

---

[6] The same is true of Ottawa, the capital city of my country, Canada. To be sure, there were important reasons other than compromise for why Canberra and Ottawa became capital cities. On the decisions in favor of Canberra and Ottawa respectively, see Davison et al. (2003) and https://prezi.com/qprau0dav7y9/why-was-ottawa-chosen-as-the-federal-capital-city/ (retrieved May 21, 2019).

them (while also indicating which philosophers have emphasized them in their work):

Disagreement (May 2015):   compromise is at issue only if there is disagreement, which there clearly was between Sydney and Melbourne.

Deadlock (Margalit 2010, 50):   the disagreement must persist so that the parties are at a deadlock, which was the case for Sydney and Melbourne; they could not agree which of them was to be the capital city.

Splitting the difference (Benjamin 1990):   to break the deadlock, the parties must decide to split the difference, and that is what the creation of Canberra did for Sydney and Melbourne. (In the continuum that lies between the conflicting parties' views, to be clear, the difference can be split at any point, not necessarily at the midpoint.)

Concession (May 2015):   in splitting the difference, the opposing parties make mutual concessions for the sake of coming to an agreement. The end result is "a concession or a deviation from what [they thought] ought to have been decided" (May 2015, 3), which was the case for Sydney and Melbourne, since neither city would be the capital.

To better understand some of these core features of standard compromises, let me explore the difference between consensus and compromise, while also asking what reasons people could have to compromise with one another given that compromise involves concession.

So, consider first how compromise differs from consensus. Both are ways of dealing with disagreement, yet each of them is unique. In coming to a consensus, opposing parties agree after persuading one another that their differences of opinion are not real or should not exist, because one (or both) parties is (or are) mistaken.[7] Through such a process, Sydney and Melbourne each could have realized that they were wrong to believe they had the best claim to being the capital city, and that the correct decision all along was to create Canberra. In that case, Canberra would be "constitutively connected" to consensus rather than compromise (Stoljar 2009). Moreover, there would have been no deadlock, no splitting of the difference (since there would have been no difference to split), and no concession. The absence of a deadlock is crucial, of course, if opposing parties are to reach a consensus: they cannot be—or see one another as—wedded to their initial positions. In the

---

[7] For simplicity, I will focus on cases that are similar to my main example in that there are only two opposing parties.

case of compromise, however, the opposite is true. Unless opposing parties take certain "differences of opinion between them as fixed" (May 2015, 4), there is no occasion for compromise.

But if the parties to a compromise continue to be wedded to their initial position, then what could motivate them to agree on a compromise? Relevant here is the fact that with compromise, the parties insist that their initial position is preferable on its merits not only to the opposing party's position, but also to any potential compromise position (May 2005). To illustrate, let:

S = the capital city should be Sydney,
M = the capital city should be Melbourne, and
C = the capital city should be Canberra.

Sydney thought that S was better on its merits than both M and C, while, Melbourne thought that M was superior on its merits. How then could both cities have agreed to C?

In short, the disagreement between Sydney and Melbourne—more importantly, their deadlock—must have given them reason to accept C and thus the creation of Canberra (May 2005, 319). Perhaps, the situation threatened something they held dear, such as peace or the new federation. At the same time, they must have thought that the other party would, in all likelihood, agree to C, for otherwise agreeing to it themselves would not have ended the deadlock and allowed them to achieve what they most wanted.[8] What motivated them to compromise, therefore, was not simply their disagreement, but the disagreement coupled with certain attitudes they held: concerning peace, for example, and what would ultimately achieve it. Together, these things would have caused them to act the way they did and made it reasonable for them to do so. Absent the initial disagreement or the supporting attitudes and there could have been no compromise.

With standard compromises, therefore, opposing parties settle their disagreement not by dissolving it—again, they take their difference of opinion

---

[8] When I return to the issue of conscientious refusals, I will focus on whether most typical objectors in reproductive health care have reasons—good ones—to cooperate with patients, not on whether they can imagine patients having good reasons to cooperate with them. It is sufficient to show that the answer to this first question is no to demonstrate that striking a good compromise between these parties is impossible.

as fixed—but by discovering reasons they have for splitting the difference in a way that both parties can accept.[9]

Now consider what makes standard compromises true or false, and good or bad. Above, I assumed that Sydney and Melbourne had reasons to agree to C. They acted based on considerations in favor of C: for instance, that C would end the deadlock, which stood in the way of the federation, which is something they wanted very much. They were not controlled instead by some external force or an internal one, such as strong feelings of fear (i.e., about an end to peace). Rather, the decision was theirs and it was reasonable from each of their perspectives. If they did in fact act in this way (reasonably), then their compromise was a true one. If instead, however, one of them—Melbourne, say—was goaded into accepting C and did so ultimately without reason, then C was a false compromise (i.e., not a compromise at all) for Melbourne. In this case, we might say that Melbourne capitulated rather than compromised (or was forced to capitulate; see Lepora 2012, 2).[10] Regardless, the solution failed to strike what was, for Melbourne, a genuine compromise. This example illustrates that whether a standard compromise is true or false depends on whether each of the opposing parties makes it for reasons, rather than having the compromise imposed on them by some external or internal power (McLeod 2008, 32).[11]

A standard compromise is good as opposed to bad if the opposing parties act for *good* reasons, rather than any old reasons. For example, Melbourne could have had a reason to accept C, but a better reason to embrace M. Perhaps the value of being the capital city was too great for it to give up on this dream without a fight. If that were the case, then we would probably say that C was not a good compromise for Melbourne although it still could have been a true compromise.

---

[9] This last point is controversial because it suggests that one party could not compromise "unilaterally" by making certain concessions, that is, without the other party reciprocating in any way (May 2015, 3). I do not exclude this possibility—perhaps there could be such one-sided compromises—but I doubt they are standard compromises.

[10] Perhaps there is a sense, however—a negative one—in which it did compromise, for we could say that it compromised (i.e., betrayed), or was forced to compromise (i.e., betray), itself (Benjamin 1990, 24).

[11] The type of reasons I'm describing here are subjective rather than objective (or motivating rather than normative, depending on how one interprets this second distinction). On such a distinction, see Alvarez (2016) (esp. section 2, "Normative Reasons"). For simplicity's sake, I have left out of the body of this chapter references to subjective versus objective reasons, because they tend to complicate rather than illuminate my analysis.

1.2 Non-standard "Third-party" Compromises

To this point, I've suggested that standard compromises have two key features: first, that the parties have met somewhere in the middle;[12] and second, that the process by which they find themselves in the middle matters to whether their compromise is true or good. Importantly, the parties to a standard compromise come to this solution with one another and without interference from a third party. Standard compromises differ in this regard from what I'll call "third-party" compromises, where a third party devises a compromise between and for the disputing parties and then imposes it on them.[13] Here are two examples of these non-standard compromises:

> A parent's two children are fighting over the last piece of cake. Knowing that the children will never work it out for themselves—they are too upset or too young for that to happen—the parent simply cuts the piece in half and gives one half to each child.

> A judge in a divorce proceeding sees that the two spouses are not able to settle their differences themselves and so decides in favour of what seems to her, the judge, to split their differences.   (Benjamin 1990, 5)[14]

Third-party compromises occur when the main parties to a dispute cannot—or cannot be relied on—to "engage in the process of compromise, [but] the situation requires a decision, and a powerful third party is able to impose a solution that seems to split the difference between them" (Benjamin 1990, 5). This sort of scenario plays out in the above examples, with the children

---

[12] Or, in the case where there are more than two parties to the compromise, they meet at some intersection point.

[13] Others have discussed compromises of this sort and referred to them simply as non-standard—or, in the case of Avishai Margalit, as "non-sanguine"—compromises (e.g., Benjamin 1990, 5–6; Margalit 2010, 53–4). They inevitably involve coercion by a third party, who makes the disputing parties compromise with one another, although as Margalit points out, the level of involvement of the third party can differ substantially; for example, this person could leave it up to the disputing parties to decide what the compromise will be or could instead develop the compromise themselves (2010, 53). I reserve the use of the term "third-party compromise" for cases where the third party's involvement is very high; this person not only demands a compromise, but also determines what it will be.

[14] The third party to a third-party compromise could, of course, be wrong about what splits the difference. To give a stark example, King Solomon's decision in the Bible literally to "split the baby" to satisfy the desires of two individuals who claimed to be the baby's parent was not a legitimate splitting of their differences (nor was it intended to be really, but rather was proposed as a way to determine who the child's true parent was; see http://www.mechon-mamre.org/p/pt/pt09a03.htm#16 (retrieved May 21, 2019). Thanks to Andrew Botterell for this example.

or the spouses as the disputing parties, and the parent or the judge as the "powerful third party." It also interestingly may describe what occurred with the creation of Canberra; the decision to create it may have been a third-party compromise, in other words, rather than the standard compromise I earlier described it to be. For according to the *Oxford Companion to Australian History*, the "founders of the Commonwealth effected a compromise" between Sydney and Melbourne; they did not achieve this outcome themselves or by themselves.[15]

The "conventional" compromise proposed for conscientious objectors in health care is also a third-party compromise. The reason is that this solution has been imposed on the parties to such conflicts by third parties, such as health policymakers and health care professional associations. For example, in Ontario, where I live, the College of Physicians and Surgeons of Ontario has required physicians who conscientiously object to providing standard services to give what it calls "effective referrals" for these services.[16] The College decided that it needed a strong policy on conscientious refusals, and could not leave it up to objecting physicians to engage in the process of compromise with their patients, presumably because of the power differential between them. So, after consulting with various groups about what its policy should be,[17] it imposed the referral requirement. Its stated goal in doing so is to "balance" the rights and interests of physicians and patients.[18] Assuming that by balancing it means compromise,[19] the College is the third party to a third-party compromise. The fact that the "conventional" compromise is a compromise of this sort explains my special interest in these non-standard compromises. Let me explore them in a bit more detail.

[15] The compromise was that "Melbourne would be the interim capital, but a site for a permanent capital would be selected by the new parliament within NSW, not less than 100 miles from Sydney" (Davison et al. 2003).

[16] On effective referrals, see the CPSO policy #2-15, "Professional Obligations and Human Rights," particularly the section "Ensuring Access to Care," at https://www.cpso.on.ca/Physicians/Policies-Guidance/Policies/Professional-Obligations-and-Human-Rights (retrieved December 18, 2019). An effective referral can be a referral to a non-objecting health care professional or to an "agency" charged with facilitating the needed referrals. By contrast, the "conventional" compromise demands the former type of action: what I have called a "proper referral." Thus, the CPSO's policy is not actually equivalent to, and is less strict than, the "conventional" compromise, which requires that objectors give referrals directly to non-objecting health care professionals. (There are also more or less strict versions of this compromise, ones that demand referrals all of the time or most of the time. I analyze a version that is less strict below.)

[17] The groups included my conscience research group. See https://www.carolynmcleod.com/policy (retrieved May 21, 2019).

[18] See note 16 and the section of the CPSO policy called "Conscience or Religious Beliefs."

[19] On the language of "balancing" vs. "compromise," see the Introduction.

With a third-party compromise, the third party devises a solution that seems to it to split the difference between the conflicting parties. An example is the parent's decision to cut the piece of cake in half. One might worry that this sort of situation does not describe a compromise at all, because the opposing parties do not in any sense compromise with one another and may not even agree with the decision that the third party makes. The children might whine and cry, for instance, when they get only half the piece of cake. To respond to this concern about third-party compromises, consider that although the warring parties may not engage in the process of compromise with one another, the third party does so in developing a solution that it believes splits the difference. There is a (forced) meeting in the middle and the process by which that happens matters, as we'll see when discussing what makes these compromises true and good.

One might persist in believing that a third-party compromise is nonsensical. But notice that if this view is correct, then the compromises proposed by compromise theorists in bioethics—including the "conventional" one—would not be compromises at all. Again, the idea with these policy solutions is not that individual health care professionals would negotiate the compromise with their patients, but rather that the compromise would be imposed on them by a third party who determines what both conscientious objectors and patients should accept as a policy solution. In short, if there was no such thing as a third-party compromise, then the work of compromise theorists would be doomed. Out of charity to them, therefore, I'll proceed on the assumption that these compromises can exist.

Like a standard compromise, a third-party compromise is genuine if it is based on reasons, and good if it is based on good reasons. The third party must choose the compromise position with these constraints in mind. This person will have to know, or assume correctly, that the opposing parties have reasons—good ones—to agree to the compromise, which is something these parties may not recognize themselves and which in turn might explain why a third party is settling their dispute.[20] For example, the minds of the spouses

---

[20] The reasons here can be either objective or subjective, while with a standard compromise, the reasons are purely subjective (see note 142). The third party could know that the opposing parties have values that give them reason to compromise with one another, in which case they have subjective reasons to do so. Alternatively, the third party could point to objective reasons for compromise, ones that are grounded in what is objectively good for each party (e.g., not being caught up in constant wrangling with one another) or in what they are objectively obligated to do. The objective reasons would still have to cohere with the initial positions of opposing parties, as I suggest in the next paragraph. They are really hybrid objective/subjective reasons. Thanks to Alida Liberman for helping me think through these points.

in divorce court could be so clouded by rage that they are unable to see they have good reasons to compromise with one another, reasons that may lie, for example, in bringing about peace with one another. Similarly, the children fighting over the piece of cake may not yet value fairness or understand what it means, yet fairness could still be a reason for compromise in their case. By cutting the cake in half, the parent could be instituting, on grounds of fairness, a compromise that is both true and good.

There may be reasons in favor of a third-party compromise that the opposing parties don't realize they have, yet the reasons still must cohere with the beliefs that caused their dispute in the first place. Third-party compromises are like standard ones in that the initial positions of the opposing parties are taken as fixed; the third party respects this difference of opinion and then develops a solution that splits it, offering reasons for accepting this solution that could exist for the opposing parties given their initial positions. The following example supports this contention. Imagine the spouses in divorce court are fighting over the custody of their children. One spouse is opposed to shared custody on the grounds that the other is a danger to their children. The judge nevertheless decides in favor of shared custody for reasons having to do with fairness and the children's welfare. It would be odd for the judge to then describe her decision as a compromise between the spouses, for there is no splitting of the difference here and the decision also requires more than just a concession on the part of the spouse who is worried about the children's safety. Instead, it demands that she give up on this perspective. That is true because fairness and the welfare of one's children are not (and could never be) reasons to share custody of one's children with someone who, by one's own lights, is a serious threat to them. The judge's decision cannot be a compromise because it does not accept this perspective.

Let me be clear that a decision in favor of shared custody in the above case could be a good one, particularly if the claim about the spouse being a threat to the children is false. My point is simply that such an outcome would not be a compromise. The reason is that with compromise—even the non-standard, third-party variety—the differing opinions of the opposing parties need to be taken as fixed. That is the case even if these opinions are incorrect or are otherwise misguided.[21] Finding reasons that do not conflict

---

[21] This point helps to explain why many of us would not want to compromise—or be the third party to a compromise—with someone who is racist (or bigoted in other ways). Doing so would require that we hold as fixed, and so basically accept for the purposes of the compromise, an initial position that is racist, and then try to split the difference between it and our own position or that of the other party. Such a demand of acceptance would be loathsome to many of us.

with them is the main task of the third party. This person needs to settle on reasons that could *be* reasons for the disputing parties given their dispute. To illustrate again, for a spouse who believes his ex is occasionally neglectful of their children rather than a serious threat to them, his love of his children and the heavy toll divorce proceedings are taking on them could be reasons to agree to shared custody, that is, if doing so would put an end to these proceedings. In the absence of reasons like these, however, the solution of shared custody could not be a compromise—which again is not to say that the solution could not be fair or good.

Let me summarize this discussion about third-party compromises. They occur when a third party to a conflict creates what seems to it to be a middle-ground solution, and then imposes this solution on the parties to the dispute. This type of compromise is genuine when it is based on reasons that actually exist for both parties, keeping in mind how they disagree with one another. The compromise is good, moreover, when it is based on good reasons. The "conventional" compromise for conscientious refusals in health care is itself a third-party compromise. The question remains, however, whether it is genuine or good.

2. Conscientious Refusals in Reproductive Health Care

Bioethicists who take the compromise approach to conscientious refusals defend policies that, in their view, amount to good and therefore true compromises for objectors. They point to reasons that they believe objectors have, as objectors, for accepting their proposed compromise. The compromise would be imposed by policymakers, making it a third-party compromise, although compromise theorists do not describe it as such (nor do they tend to distinguish between different types of compromises).

These theorists endorse a compromise solution because it is at least somewhat respectful of the conscience of health care professionals,[22] while at the same time being somewhat appreciative of the importance of patient

---

[22] That is true because of the nature of compromise (see below), but also because of the nature of conscience. According to most bioethicists writing on conscientious objection, conscience is a "subjective notion," meaning that a conscience encourages one to do what one *believes to be* morally right or wrong, and not necessarily what is objectively right or wrong (Liberman 2017, 2; see also Chapter 1). A compromise is somewhat respectful of the conscience of objectors because it takes some of their moral beliefs as fixed, allowing them ultimately to act in accordance with these beliefs.

access to care. We can see why the former would be true even when the compromise is imposed by a third party, knowing what we now know about compromises. A third-party compromise would respect the conscience of objectors to some extent because their views concerning the relevant service would be taken as fixed rather than disputed or ignored. In addition, for the compromise in question to be good, there would have to be reasons supporting it that cohere with the objectors' conscience.

This section focuses on whether reasons of this sort actually exist for typical objectors in reproductive health care: reasons that would support a good compromise for them as a solution to the conflict they have with their patients. I aim to show that in many if not most cases, the search for these reasons will be in vain. To see why, consider first that the concern of these objectors is with preventing what they perceive to be murder or the killing of what is most sacred (i.e., human life at any stage of development). Their stance is that providing the service in question (e.g., abortion or contraception) is deeply problematic because under ordinary circumstances, conduct of this sort amounts to murder (or the equivalent).[23] What possible reasons could there be for endorsing a compromise position that splits the difference between this initial position ("this is murder") and one according to which the relevant act is morally permissible ("this isn't murder at all")? Many bioethicists seem to believe there are such reasons: that typical objectors should accept. But I think this view is false, and I'll explain why using the "conventional" compromise as my central example.

2.1 The "Conventional" Compromise

Recall that according to the "conventional" compromise, health care professionals should be able to refuse to accede to a request for a service that they find morally offensive so long as they provide a referral to a health care professional who is willing and able to honor this request (Brock 2008, 194). As I noted above, this policy solution does not permit objectors to refuse to perform the service themselves in all circumstances; emergency situations are an exception to the rule that they can refuse, for example. Some bioethicists

---

[23] It is murder, that is, when it does not occur in self-defense or when the patient's life is not at stake.

  To be clear, in typical cases of conscientious objection to contraception, objectors are objecting to forms of oral contraception that they believe constitute murder, because the drugs interfere with implantation, thereby resulting in the death of a human embryo.

also recommend variations on this compromise that would occasionally allow objectors to refuse without referring their patient. Wicclair is an example (see 2011, 115).[24] I include such proposals under the banner of the "conventional" compromise, because they require objectors to give referrals most of the time.

The "conventional" compromise, though conventional (i.e., as a solution to the problem of conscientious refusals), is not obviously a good compromise. Many objectors themselves believe they have no good reason to accept it. In their view, any referral requirement makes them complicit in an act they find morally offensive (Wicclair 2011, 36; Pellegrino 2002, 239–40). For many of them, in addition, the level of complicity is so high that they would be as blameworthy for the referral as they would be for performing the offensive act themselves. This claim appears in a response made by various religious groups to a draft of the policy of the College of Physicians and Surgeons of Ontario (CPSO) that requires effective referrals. A joint submission to the College by the Christian Medical and Dental Society of Canada (CMDS) and the Canadian Federation of Catholic Physicians' Societies (CFCPS) states that for most of their members, giving a referral is no different morally speaking than committing the action themselves (Worthen 2014, 2). They liken a referral to "contracting an assassin ... [which] is morally equivalent to committing murder" (Polizogopoulos 2014, 22).[25] Anyone who reacts this strongly to the referral requirement must view the "conventional" compromise as a false compromise, that is, as a compromise that objectors have no reason to accept.[26] Alternatively, some objectors might view it simply as a bad compromise.

Whether objectors themselves believe they have reasons in favor of the "conventional" compromise, however, does not settle the question of whether

[24] To be more specific, Wicclair claims that conscientious objectors have "an obligation to *offer* to refer" their patient, particularly when they do not know whether the patient needs assistance in gaining access to the relevant service (2011, 115; his emphasis). An offer of a referral is different, of course, from an actual referral. Assuming that few patients would reject such an offer, however, Wicclair's proposal would only occasionally allow objectors to avoid providing a referral.

[25] Since the CPSO enacted its policy requiring effective referrals, the CMDS, with support from the CFCPS and some individual doctors, made an application to the Ontario Superior Court of Justice asking it to rule that the policy violates doctors' freedom of conscience (Pelley 2015). Instead, the court ruled in favor of the CPSO (*The Christian Medical and Dental Society of Canada v College of Physicians and Surgeons of Ontario*, 2018 ONSC 579).

[26] See, e.g., Polizogopoulos (2014, 21), and also the statement by the administrator of The Protection of Conscience Project on referral as a false compromise: http://www.consciencelaws.org/ethics/ethics012.aspx (retrieved May 22, 2019).

they actually have reasons to accept it. For they may have ignored certain possibilities. Indeed, compromise theorists insist there are reasons that should allow objectors to agree to the referral requirement, and I'll describe these reasons in some detail below. But first, let me emphasize that if there are such reasons, then it is not essential that objectors accept them. Rather, what is crucial is that the reasons apply to them, given their position on the service(s) in question. Once again, the "conventional" compromise is not a standard compromise, and so it isn't necessary that the parties to it understand what reasons (if any) that they have to support of it. Although compromise theorists do not acknowledge this fact, it is important to bear it in mind when discussing the reasons they offer in favor of the "conventional" compromise.

The proposed reasons include the following: 1) *respect* and *epistemic modesty* (which I will discuss together), 2) *responsibility* (more accurately, the absence of it), and 3) *professional obligation*.[27] Each of these is meant to be a reason that conscientious objectors have to accept the referral requirement. Let me describe each in turn, and then show why none of them is a reason typical objectors should accept. This analysis will draw substantially on my earlier description of the nature of compromise.[28]

2.1.1 Respect and Epistemic Modesty
Let me group respect and epistemic modesty together as Jeffrey Blustein does in the following statement:

> Respect for the moral sincerity and intelligence of others...may ground patient referral even when the referring [health care professional] believes that others are clearly in the wrong. Being convinced that one is morally in the right, moreover, is perfectly compatible with being open to the

---

[27] Also included is *liberal neutrality,* which is less promising han the others. See Blustein (1993, 310). He argues that such neutrality can give objectors—those who work in public institutions specifically—reason to endorse the "conventional" compromise. They could insist, "it is not the business of public institutions in a liberal society such as mine to enforce specific, controversial moral or religious conceptions"; these institutions should instead remain neutral on contested moral issues. With this in mind, the objector should be able to agree to the "conventional" compromise, according to Blustein (1993, 310).

But would the compromise be a good one, especially for typical objectors in reproductive health care? It would be that only if liberal neutrality could be a good reason for people to participate in what they perceive to be murder. And that's highly unlikely, since murder doesn't even fall into the category of "contested moral issues" about which a liberal institution should remain neutral. Thus, working for such an institution would not normally give objectors reason to compromise about "murderous" activities such as abortion.

[28] It also draws on McLeod (2008).

possibility that additional considerations could at some time in the future lead one to adopt and act on the position of those who presently hold an opposing moral view. (1993, 310)

The first half of this quotation mentions respect, while the second half refers to epistemic modesty (i.e., "being open to the possibility that additional considerations could at some time in the future lead one" to change one's mind). Blustein is suggesting that even for objectors who are certain about the truth of their initial position, respect and epistemic modesty can be reasons—good ones—for them to agree to a compromise that favors referrals.

Notice too that Blustein refers to "respect for the moral sincerity and intelligence of others," which can exist only in the face of *reasonable disagreement*. Similarly, epistemic modesty should not cause anyone to think that in the future, they could adopt an opposing moral view unless they perceived their disagreement with people who hold that view as reasonable. Thus, Blustein's thought, to be precise, is that respect or epistemic modesty (or both) can ground a true compromise in circumstances of reasonable disagreement. In addition, either reason could justify the "conventional" compromise when there are "other sincere and serious [health care professionals] ... [who] could do what the patient asks in good conscience," and out of respect for them or out of epistemic modesty, objectors should refer their patients to them (Blustein 310).[29]

Although Blustein's proposal may sound compelling, it is not clear to me—nor to others, most notably Simon Cabulea May (2005, 338–42)—that respect or epistemic modesty could ever be a reason for compromise.[30] Let me explain why that is true in the context first, of a standard compromise, and second, of a non-standard, third-party compromise. Recall that with a standard compromise, one continues to believe that one's initial position is superior on its merits to any other position, including the compromise one. One consequently believes that the compromise position is inferior on its merits (but worth endorsing in the circumstances). The question becomes why one would ever accept, out of respect for the sincerity or intelligence

[29] A further point Blustein could have made is that respect and epistemic modesty can support the "conventional" compromise even when objectors themselves do not view the relevant disagreement as reasonable. It could be reasonable regardless of whether they see it that way, in which case policymakers could ground the "conventional" compromise in respect or epistemic modesty.

[30] Rather than mention epistemic modesty specifically, May refers to "moral complexity" and the importance of acknowledging one's fallibility and not being dogmatic (2005, 338–9). I take this discussion to be about epistemic modesty.

of others, or because one is modest enough to know that one might be mistaken, a position that one deems to be inferior? I don't think either attitude gives one reason to agree to such a position. I can see how respect or modesty could be a reason for compromise in circumstances where it is impossible to be respectful or modest without compromising. But circumstances like these are rare, surely. Normally one can maintain that one's own position is superior to those of other people while showing respect for them (e.g., by taking their "arguments...seriously and tak[ing] the time to response to th[ose arguments] appropriately" (May 2005, 342)) or indeed while being modest (e.g., by admitting one could be wrong).

I can also see how respect or modesty could encourage one to revise one's initial position in light of others' reasonable opposition to it. But a response is a move toward consensus, not compromise. Typical objectors in reproductive health care who are epistemically modest and respect the intelligence of people who disagree with them could reverse their position on the services they object to after debating the ethics of them with others or perhaps after seeing in their own practice the negative effects on patients of not having access to these services. Because their change of heart would break the deadlock, however, between them and patients who request those services, it would remove the need for compromise. This example illustrates why respect and modesty can help to generate consensus, but not compromise.

My view about respect, modesty, and compromise extends, of course, to third-party compromises, not just to standard ones. Third parties would have to be able to assume that respect or modesty can give opposing parties reason to accept a position that is inferior on its merits to their initial positions. But then the question becomes (again), how could respect or epistemic modesty motivate anyone to endorse an inferior position? I don't think that either attitude has this power.

Not everyone will be convinced by this conclusion about respect and epistemic modesty.[31] Notice I don't need it to be true, however, to show that the compromise approach is misguided. For consider the weaker claim that neither respect nor epistemic modesty can justify the "conventional" compromise for most typical objectors in reproductive health care. To see why

---

[31] For example, one anonymous reviewer for the OUP wrote that this conclusion makes "compromise about moral issues next to impossible." I don't believe that is true, if only because the view leaves open the possibility of compromise for the sake of practical moral matters, such as peace, as we saw in the Canberra example (see May 2005). Regardless, for my purposes, I don't need to convince everyone of the conclusion I've drawn about whether respect or epistemic modesty can motivate a true compromise, as I go on to explain.

this particular claim is true, recall that the initial position of these actors is normally that the service they object to constitutes the murder (or at least unjust killing). Respect and epistemic modesty could only be a reason for them to accept the "conventional" compromise if these attitudes could give anyone reason to be complicit in murder (that is, assuming there is complicity involved in providing referrals or that many objectors reasonably believe that to be the case—but more on complicity later). It is doubtful that respect or epistemic modesty alone could provide this sort of reason, however; how could my respect for another or my epistemic modesty reasonably allow me to agree to participate in murder? The answer is that it could not. Thus, the claim that overall, one or both of these attitudes could justify the "conventional" compromise in reproductive health care contexts is misguided. This remains true even if the more general claim that these attitudes can never justify any form of compromise, in any context, is rejected.

2.1.2 Responsibility

As I have argued, it is wrongheaded to believe that respect for others or epistemic modesty could justify any sort of compromise, or at least justify the "conventional" compromise in the reproductive health care. But perhaps what is wrongheaded is the assumption that in making proper referrals for reproductive services, objectors become complicit in the provision of these services. Although many objectors contend that referrals make them complicit, they could be wrong about this fact, and some bioethicists have suggested as much. For example, Christopher Cowley says that an objector who makes a referral "is not responsible for her colleague's free actions[;] she is merely describing a fact—a widely available fact and hardly a secret—of what her colleague is willing and able to do" (2015, 362). To refuse to give a referral under these circumstances "could...be akin to sulking and preciousness," according to Cowley (362). More charitably, it would involve being mistaken, in his view, about what one is truly responsible for. If he is right about this, then the following is a reason (an objective one)[32] that objectors have to accept the "conventional" compromise: they are not responsible for what happens as a result of their referrals and so they can make them in good conscience.

To expand on Cowley, he appears to be describing what Frank Chervenak and Laurence McCullough call an "indirect referral" rather than a direct

---

[32] As noted above, reasons that can generate a third-party compromise can be objective or subjective. See note 20.

one (Chervenak and McCullough 2008; cited in Wicclair 2011, 37). The former involves simply "describing the fact" to patients that a particular colleague is willing and able to perform the service that the patient seeks and giving the patient this person's name and perhaps also their contact information. By contrast, a "direct referral" involves communicating with that colleague (directly) and overall "taking steps to assure that the patient will receive" the service in question (Wicclair 2011, 37). Like Cowley, Chervenak and McCullough don't believe there's any complicity with indirect referrals. However, they accept that there's complicity with direct referrals. Since I assume that Chervenak and McCullough's position on direct referrals is uncontroversial, let me concentrate on indirect referrals and whether it's reasonable to believe that they make one complicit.

An analysis that Wicclair gives of Chervenak and McCullough's position on indirect referrals is helpful here. Wicclair employs the following example, which he borrows from Karen Brauer, president of Pharmacists for Life (Stein 2005):

> A woman asks someone to kill her husband. The person responds that he cannot kill her husband, but he can tell her how to find someone who will. Giving the woman information that will enable her to enlist the services of a willing killer satisfies the criteria of 'indirect referral'. However, if the 'referral' results in the spouse's murder, the person who provided the information is morally complicit. Surely, that person cannot avoid complicity by claiming that the decision to kill 'is the sole province of the...[wife's] subsequent exercise of autonomy...[as Chervenak and McCullough would have it].
>
> (Wicclair 2011, 38; citing Chervenak and McCullough 2008, 232.e2)

In other words, surely, an indirect referral involves complicity. Unlike Wicclair, we *may* want to leave open the possibility that there are reasonable conceptions of responsibility or complicity according to which a person giving an indirect referral—to an assassin even—is not complicit.[33] Regardless, we should conclude from Wicclair's analysis that it is not unreasonable (to say the least) to believe that a person who provides an indirect referral

---

[33] See Liberman (2017, 8) for a discussion of how one could have a reasonable conception of responsibility and still believe there is no complicity involved in making (direct or indirect) referrals.

would be complicit (see also Liberman 2017, 8). It is also common for people to have this belief, especially when the referral is for some kind of "murderous" activity. As a result, objectors who refuse to make indirect referrals for services such as abortion are not obviously mistaken about what they are responsible for. They do not clearly have reason to accept a requirement that they offer (indirect) referrals. Cowley's statement that any opposition to this requirement "could...be akin to sulking and preciousness" is extreme (2015, 362).

On the whole, a lack of responsibility is not a reason to accept the "conventional" compromise that objectors have necessarily. They could very well *be* responsible for the actions of patients to whom they give referrals or of the colleagues that they refer patients to, either directly or indirectly.

2.1.3 Professional Obligation

Support for the referral requirement could come from other sources, however. For instance, some bioethicists insist that professional obligations, such the obligation not to abandon one's patient,[34] give objectors reason to agree to this requirement (Brock 2008; Wicclair 2011). In order to meet these obligations, objectors need—in Brock's words—either to provide "the service/product that [they] deem immoral, or instead [satisfy] the conditions of the conventional compromise" (198).

But I doubt this argument will work, again for typical objectors in reproductive health care. Consider that for many if not most of these objectors, their patient is not only the person who is or might be pregnant; instead, their patient is also the fetus in the case of a patient wanting an abortion, or the embryo that might already exist in the case of a patient seeking certain kinds of contraception. In the eyes of these objectors, their professional duties that concern patients (e.g., do not abandon them) must therefore extend to fetuses and embryos, rather than apply only to adults or children. This view about who their patients are is also implied by the initial position they have against the services that put "unborn" lives at risk. For them, providing a service such as an abortion amounts to murder, because fetuses or embryos are persons (or, at least, have moral status similar to that of persons). Moreover, if they are persons (or again, are sufficiently person-like), then it stands to reason that they are also patients. A compromise that forces objectors to reject this conclusion does not take seriously their initial

---

[34] For discussion of this obligation, see Chapter 6.

position against the services that morally offend them. The compromise could therefore not be a good one. The "conventional" compromise would be a compromise of this sort if it were grounded in a conception of professional obligation according to which fetuses and embryos are not patients. Typical objectors therefore should not, or should not necessarily, accept the "conventional" compromise on these grounds.

Perhaps this conclusion is too quick, however. For perhaps there is a professional obligation that could explain why typical objectors should accept the "conventional" compromise even though (or if) they view fetuses and embryos as patients. Consider the duty of care that health care professionals have to their patients, which could provide these objectors with a reason to offer referrals. This duty could permit those who morally object to abortion, for example, to refer patients seeking an abortion to a competent abortion provider, because otherwise the patients might seek out an incompetent provider or try to abort themselves. And if they did that, then *both* they and the fetus would suffer. In this way, the duty of care supports the "conventional" compromise.

The soundness of the above reasoning depends on how likely it is that conscientiously denying the referral would cause the harm I just described. It may be that the patient requesting the abortion could get a safe abortion quite easily without assistance from the objecting professional. In circumstances like these, there is actually a strong reason *against* providing a referral, assuming that the near certainty the fetus will die if the objector gives the referral outweighs the mere possibility that both patients will die, or be maimed or hurt, if the objector refuses to do so.[35]

In short, although it is possible that professional obligation, in particular the duty of care, could ground the "conventional" compromise in some

---

[35] Notice that one could run a similar argument about other reproductive services, such as in vitro fertilization. Health care professionals who morally object to IVF because of the likelihood that embryos will be killed in the process might think that they should provide referrals for IVF to fertility specialists who will not over-stimulate patients' ovaries. Over-stimulation puts patients' health at risk and can result in the creation—and ultimate destruction—of many embryos. Better that the patients receive a referral from them rather than end up with a specialist who is cavalier about the creation of human embryos.

As with the reasoning about referrals for abortion, however, the above reasoning is sound only if it is *likely* that the proposed harm will occur if the objectors refuse to refer. But this outcome is unlikely in areas where fertility specialists tend to act responsibly or are well regulated: in other words, where chances are good that patients who seek out a fertility specialist on their own will find one who takes the duty of care seriously. I take it that such areas are common (at least outside of countries like the United States where assisted reproduction tends to be poorly regulated).

circumstances, it is unlikely to do so in many cases involving typical refusals. A background assumption here is that in taking the compromise approach, we must regard as fixed objectors' positions on controversial reproductive services, positions that extend not only personhood but also patienthood to embryos and fetuses. Yet once we do that, we will hard pressed to find a professional obligation that could justify these professionals splitting the difference with their patients (i.e., those who make the requests that offend against their conscience).

Professional obligation is but one of the reasons I've examined for why typical objectors in reproductive health care might accept the "conventional" compromise, the other reasons being respect, epistemic modesty, and not being responsible for the consequences of a referral. I have argued that either these are not reasons at all for why objectors should agree to the "conventional" compromise or they are not *good* reasons for them to do so (not necessarily anyway). The third parties to this compromise cannot assume otherwise, which becomes clear once we reflect on the nature of the relevant objections (typical ones in reproductive health care), but also on the nature of compromises and what it means for them to be both genuine and good.

Let me emphasize that my argument does not exclude the possibility that some objectors—even typical ones in reproductive health care—could accept the "conventional" compromise. Some might interpret the services they object to or interpret, say, moral responsibility or professional obligation, in a way that allows them to endorse this solution. If so, wonderful! For then the requirement that they give proper referrals would sit well with them and their conscience. I have claimed that for many if not most typical objectors, this requirement will, however, be seriously problematic. They will have no reason, or no good reason, to consent to it, mainly because of how strong their objections are. The "conventional" compromise does not amount to a good compromise for them.

If I am correct, then the "conventional" compromise does not do what compromise theorists want it to do: namely, promote the interests of both patients and objectors to some degree. What about other possible compromises? Those who support the compromise approach could develop alternatives to the "conventional" compromise, as some have done (e.g., Lynch 2008). My worry, however, is that no such attempt will succeed for typical refusals, because of how strongly the objectors in these cases oppose the relevant services (e.g., abortions). Alternatively, I suspect that if the proposed compromise is good for these objectors, then it is bad for patients. To explain this last point, for a compromise to be an improvement on the "conventional" one from objectors' perspectives, it would have to give them more freedom of conscience. But the more freedom they have in this regard, the worse things get for patients. Consider Lynch's institutional compromise, which I outlined in Chapter 3. Her solution amounts to a compromise for objectors insofar as it requires them to make the concession of fulfilling "nonnegotiable duties" (e.g., informing patients of all of their treatment options and giving care in emergencies), that is, regardless of whether performing these duties violates their conscience. Beyond that, however, Lynch believes that physicians should be able to conduct their practice as they morally see fit, and the institution of the licensing board should be responsible for matching patients with physicians whose moral values allow them to perform the treatment that patients need. Importantly, on this account, objecting physicians do not have a duty to provide referrals for services they morally object to. This "institutional" compromise may be good for objectors, but as I argued in Chapter 3, it is bad for patients if only because it threatens their ability to trust in health care professionals and professions. Patients should therefore reject Lynch's institutional compromise, since it is not a good compromise for them. Again, I am skeptical that bioethicists could come up with a compromise that is good, generally speaking, for *both* patients and objectors.

3. Conclusion

How the compromise approach could work for typical refusals in reproductive health care therefore remains mysterious to me. I have argued that for a solution to these conflicts to count as a good compromise, it would have to be supported by reasons that take the nature of the conflict seriously and that are stronger than the reasons both parties would have to refuse to make any concessions. Because of the strength of the moral convictions of most typical objectors, however, it is unlikely that such a solution exists. Using the "conventional" compromise as my primary example, I have tried to show that the third parties to this solution will be hard pressed to justify it as a good or even a true compromise for many (or most) objectors. To be clear, my point is not that this compromise is a bad one for *patients*; indeed, I think the opposite is the case. The problem is that there is no symmetrical argument for the other side; the "conventional" compromise is not a good compromise for many objectors.

If the compromise approach is doomed, particularly when it comes to typical refusals in reproductive health care, then we need to find an alternative approach. We need to do that for developing not only policies that are specific to these refusals but also ones that are general or meant to apply to all conscientious refusals. The reason, again, has to do with how common typical refusals are (see the Introduction); if a general policy cannot work for them, then it cannot be a good policy on conscientious refusals. In what follows, I argue that a general policy informed by my "prioritizing approach" can work for typical refusals, and even for atypical ones.

5

Fidelity to Patients

The most vexing problem posed by conscientious refusals in health care is how to justify appropriate regulations on them. I argued in Chapter 4 that the popular strategy of striking a compromise between conscientious objectors and patients will not work for many if not most typical refusals in reproductive health care. It therefore should not inform policies on these refusals specifically, or on conscientious refusals generally, because of how common typical refusals are. The consequence is that we need a different approach to regulating conscientious refusals in health care.

The alternative to the compromise approach is to prioritize one set of interests over the other: that is, the objector's moral integrity (see Chapter 1) over the moral identity, sense of security, autonomy, and trust of the patient (see Chapters 2 and 3), or vice versa. Such an avenue is distinct from compromise because it does not require that we accommodate both sets of interests to some extent.[1] (At the same time, it does not preclude us from doing so). Since with many typical refusals, it is difficult, if not impossible to advance both sets of interests simultaneously, some kind of prioritizing approach must be preferable to the compromise one.

We could have regulations that prioritize the moral integrity of objectors, although that would be a mistake, in my view.[2] If we interpret moral integrity as I did in Chapter 1, then this interest amounts to objectors acting on their best (secular or religious) moral judgment, but not necessarily doing what is morally correct. Such conduct also has both personal and social value; it allows objectors to lead authentic moral lives, and at the same, to contribute to social debate about what is morally worth doing (see Chapter 1). Although these personal and social interests may be substantial, I think prioritizing them over patients' interests—and therefore having unrestricted conscientious

---

[1] In particular, unlike with compromise, we needn't find reasons that both parties could have to accept our policy solution, while holding divergent positions on the service in question. See Chapter 4.

[2] Wicclair calls this approach "conscience absolutism." For more discussion about why it is problematic, see his Chapter 2 (2011).

Conscience in Reproductive Health Care: Prioritizing Patient Interests. Carolyn McLeod, Oxford University Press (2020).
© Carolyn McLeod.
DOI: 10.1093/oso/9780198732723.001.0001

objection in health care—is seriously problematic. Consider that by doing so, we would not be guaranteeing moral objectivity. Instead, we would almost certainly be allowing harm, that is, to patients (see Chapters 2 and 3), and by someone who has a professional duty not to harm them. Consider as well that objectors could satisfy the social interest we have in them (or anyone) acting on their best moral judgment by rallying outside of the clinic or hospital in favor of policy change in health care.[3] Indeed, they could further this social interest more by making their objections public in this way rather than by objecting privately in their health care practices.

The above points about harm to patients and the professional duty of objectors suggest that a strategy of prioritizing *patients'* interests—and therefore prohibiting or at least severely restricting conscientious objection—*is* plausible. I call this approach "*the* prioritizing approach,"[4] because it is the only one of its kind that is a serious contender to the compromise approach. Assuming I am right about this fact, the question remains, however: on what grounds can the interests of patients be prioritized over those of objectors?

In answering this question, I have looked for guidance in the literature on fiduciaries, and on health care professionals as fiduciaries. This is an obvious place to turn because of the emphasis there on a duty of loyalty to patients (more generally, to beneficiaries), which involves prioritizing their interests over one's own interests. The literature on health care professionals as fiduciaries focuses almost exclusively on physicians. It also reveals that the claim that physicians are fiduciaries, or ought to be regarded as such, is contentious. Even more contentious, I assume, is the idea that other gatekeepers to controversial reproductive services are fiduciaries (e.g., pharmacists or nurse practitioners). As noted in the Introduction, I want to focus on health care professionals who serve this gatekeeping role—who are meant to control access to the relevant services by deciding who should have it—because their conscientious refusals can seriously disrupt access. (For simplicity, throughout, I use the term "health care professional" to refer only to these professionals.) I will defend the claim that they are fiduciaries, at least while acting in their gatekeeping capacity, and will go on to

---

[3] As I discuss in Chapter 6, however, there may be ethical limitations on such behavior that require the objectors to act not as health care professionals but as private persons when they are striving to make policy change.

[4] The approach supports what Wicclair calls "the incompatibility thesis," which is that conscientious objection is incompatible with one's professional duty (2011, Ch. 2). Wicclair rejects this view on the grounds that no theory of health professional obligation can back it up, although he fails to consider a theory according to which health care professionals are fiduciaries to their patients (2011, 44–85). I defend the prioritizing approach using this kind of account.

use the fiduciary model of the patient–health care professional relationship to argue in favor of the prioritizing approach to conscientious refusals.

The argument in this chapter is somewhat limited in scope. It discusses cases of conscientious refusal where there is an existing (fiduciary) relationship between the objector and the patient. The focus is on what health care professionals are obligated to do when they are inside such a relationship and conscientiously object to what *their* patients request of them. By contrast, Chapter 6 deals with obligations of conscientious objectors that might exist outside of such a relationship, including duties to enter relationships with patients whose values conflict with their own.

This chapter has three main sections. Section 1 explains briefly what philosophers or bioethicists have said in favor of prioritizing patient interests in the context of conscientious refusals. I am not alone in taking what I've called the prioritizing approach, although I do defend it in a unique way. Section 2 clarifies what it means to say that physicians and other health care professionals are (or ought to be regarded as) fiduciaries, along with why they are indeed fiduciaries, in certain contexts at least. This section also discusses the primary duty of fiduciaries, which is that of loyalty. Finally, Section 3 defends the prioritizing approach to conscientious refusals using the fiduciary model of the patient–health care professional relationship. I contend that this model alone cannot tell us why this approach is justified, and so I supplement it with other insights about conscientious refusals, many of which come from previous chapters. This discussion initially follows the pattern of those earlier chapters in concentrating on typical refusals in reproductive health care. But then it departs from this pattern by examining briefly *atypical* refusals, including (but not limited to) those that many people—regardless of their moral stance on abortion—would claim are morally *appropriate*. (A putative example is a refusal to perform a sex-selective abortion where these abortions are legal, professionally accepted, and yet normally target female fetuses.) The goal is to show that the prioritizing approach can work not only for typical refusals, but also for atypical ones. It can—and indeed should, in my opinion—inform policies on conscientious refusals that are general, rather than specific to typical refusals.

1. Consent, Being "My Profession's Keeper," and Fair Play

A number of theorists have taken a strong stand against conscientious refusals in health care (e.g., Kolers 2014; Kelleher 2010; Card 2007; Savulescu 2006;

Savulescu and Schuklenk 2017). They insist that health care professionals[5] do not have a right of conscientious refusal—that those who have conscientious objections must prioritize the interests patients have in receiving standard services over their own interest in preserving their conscience. While they give different sorts of reasons for their view—including that too much conscientious refusal is burdensome for patients (Savulescu 2006; Kelleher 2010) or that the content of certain objections is morally or epistemologically problematic (Card 2007)—I want to concentrate on reasons that concern the duties health care professionals have qua health care professional. Like me, most of these authors contend that these professionals have role-related duties that conflict with them being conscientious objectors.

Let me focus in this literature on the work of Paul Kelleher and Avery Kolers, since they offer the most sustained explanations for why health care professionals, qua professional, should not have a right to conscientious refusal. The reasons these philosophers give, respectively, include consent—for example, to offering standard services—and the importance of being a "keeper" of one's profession. I will also consider an additional reason—fair play—which Elizabeth Fenton and Loren Lomasky use to defend a moderate position on conscientious refusal, but which could easily support the "immoderate" positions that Kelleher, Kolers, and I endorse (Fenton and Lomasky 2005).[6] I will describe each of these reasons in turn—consent, being "my profession's keeper," and fair play—and then explain why I find each of them wanting and why I prefer a different sort of explanation for why health care professionals should not be permitted to make conscientious refusals (within established relationships with patients, at least).[7]

Turning first to Kelleher, he claims that by voluntarily assuming their professional role, health care professionals consent to doing what the role

---

[5] These authors tend to focus on either physicians or pharmacists, although their reasons apply equally well to all health care professionals. Some of them also concentrate on refusals that target a specific kind of service (e.g., emergency contraception; Card 2007 and Kelleher 2010), though much of their reasoning applies to other refusals as well. When discussing their theories, I will therefore refer simply to health care professionals making conscientious refusals.

[6] Indeed, some bioethicists have suggested that it could be used in this way (e.g., Savulescu and Schuklenk 2017, 2). On Fenton and Lomasky's argument, see Chapter 2.

[7] A further explanation is that health care professionals who identify with their social role have enough of a reason to do what the role requires that they should act this way. The reason stems from the fact that being in the role gives their life meaning and promotes their autonomy (Sciaraffa 2009). Such an argument is limited unfortunately to cases involving professionals who identify with their social role and identify with it more than they identify with being, say, Christian or pro-life about abortion.

requires, which in turn makes them duty-bound to deliver standard services, even when their conscience prohibits it. In Kelleher's words, a health care professional could not insist that she is being "deprive[d] of adequate freedom to express her religious convictions, or to act on her conscience, if a job she voluntarily pursues or holds—to the exclusion of many other viable career paths—requires her to dispense" a particular medication or offer a particular service (2010, 301).

Kolers, by contrast, presents an argument based on the social value that health care professions have (2014).[8] Preserving them requires that individual members are "keepers" of their profession, adhering to its norms and objectives, rather than to personal conscience. Kolers refers to the important aims that a profession like medicine has, and how achieving them requires a "confluence of aims" amongst individual members (4). Collectively, these individuals must serve their profession's purpose(s)—their actions must be coordinated in this way—for otherwise, there could be no profession. For Kolers, what is at stake in allowing health care professionals to listen to their conscience, whatever it may say to them, is the very existence of their profession.[9]

A further reason one might give for why health care professionals are obligated not to be conscientious objectors concerns fair play. Considering the many benefits that they receive in becoming or simply being health care professionals—the subsidized education, the prestige (especially for physicians), and the monopoly or guild-like status "conferred on their profession by the state" (Kelleher 2010, 297)—it's only fair that they always perform their professional duties. Although one might have to do quite a bit of work to explain why that's fair, an argument like this could succeed. Still, it's not the line of argument I want to take. Neither do I want to rely on consent or being "my profession's keeper." Here's why, in brief.

What is most troublesome, for me at least, about conscientious refusals is that the objectors tend to misuse or abuse the power they have over patients. That is true with typical objections in reproductive health care or really with any objections where professionals refuse to accede to patients' autonomous

---

[8] He specifically rejects what he calls the "Consent model" of role obligations (2–4), and defends instead what he terms "Professionalism." My own theory is a version of Professionalism, insofar as professionals are fiduciaries. See Bayles (1988).

[9] In summarizing his position, he writes: a "profession that genuinely serves the public good...is a fragile and hard-won achievement"; "preserving [it]...is the responsibility of all who practice a profession" (2014, 7).

requests for standard services.[10] The reasons just discussed do not refer to this sort of problem, however. In general, they focus too much on the health care professionals themselves (what *they* have consented to, how *they* benefit) or the profession itself (*its* preservation, *its* value), and not enough on what health care professionals do to patients when they conscientiously refuse to provide them with standard services.

A further concern, specifically about consent, is that this reason may not preclude all or even most conscientious refusal. In particular, where the profession or the state is very permissive toward conscientious refusal in health care—there may be laws in place that require them to be this way—individual health care professionals have not consented to adhere to their profession's norms or objectives, regardless of what their conscience dictates. In that case, there is no consent they have given that prohibits them from conscientious refusing to heed patients' requests for standard services.

To summarize, I want to take a strong stand against conscientious refusals—especially typical ones—based on what health care professionals are required to do as health care professionals. In that sense, my position is similar to that of other philosophers, including Kelleher and Kolers. But I don't think the justifications they offer necessarily support such a stand or support it in a way that focuses enough attention on patient interests. To expand briefly on this last point, these authors take a position that amounts, in the end, to patients' interests being prioritized over objectors' interests, but they (the authors) do not prioritize patient interests when reasoning for their point of view. Since I want to be able to reason in this way and strongly suspect that by adopting a fiduciary model of the patient-health care professional relationship, I will be able to do so, let me turn now to a discussion about fiduciaries.

2. Fiduciaries, Fidelity, Physicians, and Pharmacists

It is common for bioethicists to say about patient–*physician* relationships that they are fiduciary. Yet rarely do they define what this means. What is a

---

[10] It is not obviously true of conscientious objections where the patient agrees (or would agree) with the objector's view that the standard service is immoral. Sometimes health care professionals refuse to abide by what they deem to be an unjust law or policy and their patients are happy about this fact. I discuss cases like these in both the Introduction and the Conclusion. They involve what I and others call "conscientious commitment," rather than "conscientious refusal." Since the latter (conscientious refusal) is the focus of this book, the former is beyond the scope of it.

fiduciary relationship? The answer is that it is both a "distinctive type of legal relationship" and a relationship of power (i.e., relationship in which one party has power over another; Miller 2011, 235). Let me highlight what is special about it in terms of power. I will then explain why fidelity is morally crucial in a fiduciary relationship, and will finally turn to whether, or when, health care professionals are fiduciaries. This last part will focus primarily on physicians and pharmacists, although I will extend my argument to other gatekeepers of reproductive services like abortions.

2.1 Fiduciaries

Since the fiduciary relationship is a distinctive kind of legal relationship, I take my cue from legal theorists in defining it, especially from Paul Miller but also from Lionel Smith (2014). That said, I am interested in this relationship's *moral* dimensions, and will later make moral claims (and moral claims only) about fiduciary obligations. Miller and Smith define the fiduciary relationship, or what it is to be a fiduciary, against a backdrop of substantive disagreement in law on such topics (see, e.g., Gold and Miller 2014). Since their theories ring true, however, to how the courts (see esp. Miller 2011), other legal theorists (see, e.g., Gold and Miller 2014), and professional ethicists (e.g., Bayles 1988) view the fiduciary relationship, I believe they have captured what is central to it.

Miller distinguishes the fiduciary relationship by the type of power that fiduciaries possess:

i) Power that is discretionary—there is "scope for judgment in the exercise of it" (Miller 2011, 273)—as opposed to bare power, such as that of a crossing guard to get the traffic to stop.

ii) Power in the form of authority rather than mere influence or control (Miller 2011, 272); for example, a person who stages an intervention into the life of an addict/friend is not authorized to do so, whereas fiduciaries are authorized—normally by beneficiaries themselves through their consent—to act in their beneficiary's best interests.

iii) Authority over the "significant practical interests" of the beneficiary, rather than any old interests (Miller 2011, 276). Significant practical interests are those interests that one promotes or protects when exercising a legal capacity, such as the capacity to "make decisions relating to [someone's] health and personal welfare" and "to license...access

to, contact with, or use of, [someone's] physical person or property"
(Miller 2014, 71). The interests are significant in that some serious legal
matter is at stake, and practical because they can be affected by the
exercise of a legal capacity. Interests over which, say, a personal trainer
or a plumber has power generally do not meet this standard.

Unlike crossing guards or personal trainers, people such as trustees, corporate directors, and lawyers are fiduciaries. As such, they have a distinctive
form of power. To quote Miller, they have "discretionary authority to set or
pursue [significant] practical interests...of another" (2011, 278). To quote
Smith, fiduciaries are "empowered to exercise decision-making authority on
behalf of another" (2014, 608). The fiduciary relationship is importantly a
relationship in which one party acts on the other's behalf.[11]

Since bioethicists tend to conflate fiduciary relationships with trust
relationships,[12] let me describe briefly how the two are different. While
most fiduciary relationships are, in fact, trust relationships, the latter category is broader. For instance, the addict probably trusts the intervention-
ist/friend as a friend. And if that is true, then the friend has discretionary
power, which is a central feature of trust or, more accurately, of being trusted
(Baier 1986, esp. 237–9). Since the friend lacks discretionary *authority*,
however, to stage the intervention, he is not a fiduciary in this context.
Trusted individuals do not all possess the same kind or degree of power that
fiduciaries do.

A further feature of a fiduciary relationship is the vulnerability of the
beneficiary. In describing this characteristic, Miller distinguishes between
two types of vulnerability: that which is extrinsic to the fiduciary relationship and therefore "circumstantial," and that which is intrinsic to this relationship and therefore "structural" (Miller 2011, 254, 279). (The latter hinges on
"structural qualities of the fiduciary relationship"; 279.) Not all beneficiaries
experience circumstantial vulnerability, though many do as a result, for
example, of poverty or oppression. But all beneficiaries experience structural
vulnerability, since all are subject to a fiduciary's discretionary authority and

---

[11] Of course, not all relationships in which one party acts on behalf of the other are fiduciary. On these relationships in general, see Howard 2013.

[12] For example: "the classical axiom of medicine since Hippocratic times—'To help or at
least to do no harm'—makes trust on the part of the patient the central requirement of the
fiduciary relationship" (Zaner 1991, 47); and "trust has special moral dimensions which are the
foundation for professional ethics, what Barber has called 'fiduciary relationships'" (Pellegrino
1991, 72).

are at risk of its abusive exercise. What beneficiaries are vulnerable to, specifically, is the abuse or misuse of fiduciary power. Usually, they cannot protect themselves against this threat, because they lack the knowledge or skill necessary to be able to assess whether the fiduciary is indeed acting in their interests.[13] This fact helps to explain both the vulnerability of the beneficiary *and* the power of the fiduciary.

The discretionary authority of fiduciaries is substantial, yet at the same time, it is limited (Miller 2011, 275). For example, fiduciaries are normally authorized to act on the beneficiary's behalf only within a certain sphere, such as that of the beneficiary's finances or health. They are presumed to have specialized knowledge or expertise in this area, which helps to clarify both why they are granted the authority in the first place and what the limits of this authority are (Miller 2011, 283). (Its limits match those of the fiduciary's presumed expertise.) Fiduciaries are also authorized to make decisions for beneficiaries that serve the beneficiaries' ends, not the fiduciary's own personal ends. Fiduciary authority is limited in this second respect as well.

In sum, the fiduciary relationship involves a distinctive kind of power: that is, authority to set or promote significant practical interests of another, usually within a certain sphere. This power engenders a certain type of vulnerability: structural vulnerability to the misuse or abuse of discretionary authority over one's significant practical interests.

2.2 Fidelity

The primary fiduciary duty is one of loyalty or fidelity to one's beneficiary.[14] This obligation requires that fiduciaries devote themselves to serving their beneficiaries' interests within the sphere of the authority that is vested in them. They therefore, in this sphere, must take care to avoid as much as possible conflicts between their interests and those of their beneficiaries, and between their obligations to beneficiaries and their obligations to others (Miller 2011, 257). (These are the "no conflict rules" in fiduciary law: no

---

[13] Even if they could monitor the fiduciary in this way, however, because they had the relevant knowledge or skill, they could not do so while being in a fiduciary relationship with this person. The reason is that fiduciaries need room to exercise the discretion that is essential to their role as fiduciaries.

[14] Specialists in fiduciary law generally agree on this point. They disagree over other duties, however, including a duty of care; Miller writes, it "is...unclear whether the duty of care, which requires fiduciaries to act reasonably in fulfilling their mandates, is a fiduciary duty" (2013, 976; citing, e.g., Conaglen 2010).

conflicts of interest or obligation.) There are both conceptual and moral reasons for the requirement of loyalty. Let me explain.

Conceptually, for fiduciaries to be acting on behalf of their beneficiaries, they must be pursuing the interests of their beneficiaries rather than their own interests or other interests. This point comes from Smith. He uses the following analogy to argue that one does not act on someone else's behalf if one acts simply out of self-interest:

> Albert and Belinda are playing backgammon, and Belinda is called away to the telephone. The call takes longer than expected; Albert becomes impatient; Belinda calls out, 'Play my turn for me.' Albert rolls the dice and, like a fiduciary, is presented with a range of possible moves. The only way to make sense of the idea of Albert playing Belinda's turn for her is that he must play it in the way that he thinks is in her best interests. Of course, he might deliberately make what he thinks is a bad move, but this would not count as playing her turn for her, in line with the authority that she gave. Like the disloyal exercise of a fiduciary power, it would amount to a misuse of authority.   (2014, 613)

Surely, Smith is right that we act on someone's behalf only if we act in that person's interests, which in turn involves acting in accordance with what the person has authorized us to do. This logic is relevant to fiduciaries if a fiduciary is indeed someone who acts on behalf of another. The grounds for the fiduciary duty of loyalty lie within that conception.

But there are also important moral (as opposed to conceptual) reasons one could give for the duty of loyalty. One could insist, for example, that loyalty is the appropriate moral response when others are vulnerable to discretionary authority that one possesses over them. Miller takes this sort of line. He says that the duty of loyalty "responds to and reflects a *kind of vulnerability* peculiar to the fiduciary relationship; namely, the inherent susceptibility of the beneficiary to exploitative exercise of discretionary power by the fiduciary" (Miller 2011, 280; his emphasis). Although Miller emphasizes vulnerability in this statement, what is equally if not more important, morally speaking, is exploitation: more specifically, the beneficiary's susceptibility to it. Beneficiaries are at serious risk of exploitation by fiduciaries: that is, of fiduciaries taking unfair advantage of them in their vulnerable state (McLeod and Baylis 2007, 475; citing Sample 2003; see also Zwolinski and Wertheimer 2016). That is true because of the knowledge gap between them and their fiduciaries, and also because of the discretion fiduciaries have. The knowledge gap makes it all too easy for fiduciaries to convince beneficiaries that a certain course of action advances their interests, when objectively speaking it does not. In addition, the discretion fiduciaries have in deciding how to advance their beneficiaries' interests gives them room to convince *themselves* that they are furthering these interests, when instead they are promoting their own interests or those of a third party. This last point helps to explain not only the risk of exploitation in the fiduciary relationship but also the rule that fiduciaries avoid conflicts of interest.[15]

Thus, one can explain the fiduciary duty of loyalty in moral terms by pointing to the vulnerability of the beneficiary, or more specifically to what the beneficiary is vulnerable to (i.e., exploitation). Alternatively, one could try to give a contractual argument for this duty, as some authors do in the literature on fiduciaries.[16] One could claim, in other words, that the duty is a product of an agreement (implicit or explicit) between the parties to the fiduciary relationship. Could it be that, however, a simple matter of agreement? I don't think so. The reason is that regardless of what two parties agree to, if one of them has acquired discretionary authority over significant practical interests of the other, then the first party must be loyal to the other in exercising this authority (Smith 2014). Otherwise, this person would be subjecting the other to a substantial risk of exploitation, which itself is morally problematic. It follows that what grounds the duty of loyalty is not consent, but the very nature of the fiduciary relationship. Moreover, fiduciaries have the duty regardless of whether they consent to it.[17]

Let me be clear that the fiduciary duty of loyalty does not require that fiduciaries ignore their own interests. The duty demands only that they

[15] Smith writes, "[a] conflict of interest arises when a person is required to exercise judgement in an unselfish way, but is in a position in which that judgement is liable to be affected by self-regarding or otherwise conflicting considerations...When a person exercises judgement in a conflict situation, it is impossible for that person to be certain that they have excluded extraneous considerations" (2014, 624). See also Samet (2008).

[16] See, e.g., Easterbrook and Fischel (1991), and Langbein (1995), cited in Laby (2008).

[17] As Smith puts it, the "requirement of loyalty is inherent in [this] relationship." Therefore, one needn't presume that fiduciaries are in these relationships voluntarily to find them in breach of the duty of loyalty (Smith 2014, 614).

Although consent (or contract) cannot explain the duty of loyalty, it could influence what the duty requires: more specifically, whether it requires that the fiduciary avoid *all* conflicts of interest. (On whether it demands that they avoid all conflicts of obligation, see Section 2.3.) The possibility exists in law for the parties to a fiduciary relationship to agree that the one will act for the other despite having certain conflicts of interest (see, e.g., Samet 2008, 771; Harding 2016, 81–3). Fiduciaries must still act in beneficiaries' interests in the face of these conflicts, however, for otherwise they would violate their duty of loyalty. Presumably, the law justifies this exception to the no-conflict rule because the fiduciaries are open about their conflicts and their beneficiaries agree to them, thereby lowering the risk of exploitation substantially.

promote relevant interests of their beneficiary—those relevant to the sphere of their authority over the beneficiary—and that they not act on interests of their own (or others) that conflict with these interests. There is scope here for fiduciaries to act self-interestedly, to be sure. They could do so while acting in the relevant interests of their beneficiary if the two actions are compatible with one another. For example, they could have a colleague cover for them while they are on holiday, which should satisfy their beneficiary's interests (in the short-term at least), along with their need to have some time off.

In this brief discussion about fiduciaries and fidelity, I have followed Smith and Miller respectively in grounding the fiduciary duty of loyalty in our conception of the fiduciary as someone who acts on behalf of another and in the structural vulnerability of the beneficiary to the exploitative use of fiduciary power. These arguments make the duty dependent on structural aspects of the fiduciary relationship, rather than on any sort of agreement between the parties. The duty requires that fiduciaries prioritize relevant interests of their beneficiaries over their own interests when the two conflict with one another, and more generally, to be focused on pursuing these interests of beneficiaries (e.g., health care or legal interests).

2.3 Physicians

As I've noted, it is common for bioethicists to claim that physicians are fiduciaries. I am now in a position to explain what that means. Physicians are fiduciaries because they have discretionary authority to act on behalf of their patients in a certain sphere—that of their health—and patients are vulnerable to them exploiting this power. This relationship engenders a duty of loyalty in physicians, that is, a duty to put their patients' health interests first, ahead of their own interests. Other health care professionals are in the same sort of position relative to their patients, at least when they are acting as the gate-keepers to reproductive health services, or so I will argue. But let me begin with physicians, since there is considerably more literature on them as fiduciaries, and starting with them should smooth the way toward establishing that other health care professionals are (or at least can be) fiduciaries.

I suspect many bioethicists will find the fiduciary model of the patient–physician relationship attractive (especially in contrast to the contract model, which defines the relationship entirely in terms of a contract; see Veatch 1991). One reason why is that the fiduciary model highlights the inequality of power in the relationship and the vulnerability of patients to the misuse or abuse of this power by physicians. A second reason concerns the idea that physicians have some duties to patients (one at least: loyalty) that arise out of their power relationship, not out of any sort of agreement between the parties. This idea should be both familiar and compelling: familiar, because feminist ethicists (among others) have made similar claims about responsibilities in relationships (e.g., Kittay 1999; Walker 1998; Whitbeck 1983); and compelling, because the view suggests that physicians cannot negotiate their way out of doing all that they owe to patients. Physicians cannot strike morally binding agreements with patients, in other words, that would permit them to focus on their own interests rather than on patient interests.

Though attractive, the fiduciary model of the patient-physician relationship is contentious, as I've said. Two main objections to it appear in the literature: one concerning loyalty and the other, paternalism (Ryman 2017). The first objection is that physicians are seriously limited in how devoted they can be to one patient's interests, because they are required to have multiple loyalties. They must act on behalf of numerous parties: patients (plural), hospitals they work for, the public (e.g., in reigning in health care spending or protecting people from infectious or otherwise dangerous patients), etc. (Criddle and Fox Decent 2018). This fact puts "a strain" on the fiduciary picture of the patient–physician relationship (Rodwin 1995).

To respond to this objection, the strain is serious only if the multiple loyalties of physicians are frequently divided (Ryman 2017). Many fiduciaries have multiple loyalties; for example, parents are fiduciaries to their children and many parents have more than one child. Yet they do not cease to be fiduciaries because of this fact, which would be true as well of physicians (Criddle and Fox Decent 2018). The important question is whether physicians frequently experience *divided* loyalties. Emma Ryman suggests, rightly I think, that if they do experience that because of the demands of health care systems, then the complaint should be with these systems, not with the fiduciary model. The alternative is an unhappy one: that we accept that physicians can use their power to serve interests other than those of their patients.

A second objection to the fiduciary model is that it doesn't fit with the modern bioethical requirement that physicians respect the autonomy of their patients. Such a concern exists insofar as the fiduciary relationship is paternalistic, which some claim that it is. Since this objection is somewhat complicated, let me explain it in some detail. I'll then defend the fiduciary model against it using an understanding of patient autonomy that I believe many bioethicists share.

Perhaps unsurprisingly given the nature of the fiduciary relationship, some view it as paternalistic. Daniel Markovits writes, for example: "the beneficiary has sought...the fiduciary's independent and...unreviewable judgment, and thus also the paternalism that the exercise of this judgment inevitably involves" (2014, 217; cited in Ryman 2017, Ch. 1). Smith says that with the acquisition of discretionary authority comes a "partial transfer of autonomy," which suggests some degree of paternalism (2014, 613). The position represented here—what I will call "Fiduciary Paternalism"—is that paternalism is inherent to the fiduciary relationship.[18]

Fiduciary Paternalism creates a problem for the fiduciary model of the patient–physician relationship, because this relationship is meant to be non-paternalistic, specifically where patients are competent to make decisions about their own health care. Bioethicists have roundly criticized medical paternalism with such patients (and also with those who have family or friends who can serve as substitute decision-makers for them). One reason is that patients can have values, experiences, or just lives that differ substantially from those of physicians and that make it reasonable for patients to make choices about their health that their physician would not recommend for them (McCullough and Wear 1985, 302). To put the point a little differently, physicians are often not well-placed to decide on their own what is in patients' best interests, and that is especially true—as feminist bioethicists have insisted (see esp. Sherwin 1998)—for patients who occupy very different social locations than most physicians do.[19]

To remedy the problem that Fiduciary Paternalism poses for the fiduciary model of the patient–physician relationship, I want to reject Fiduciary Paternalism.[20] My view, in short, is that when fiduciaries exercise authority granted to them by competent beneficiaries to use their best judgment to pursue interests the beneficiaries have established for themselves, they—the fiduciaries—do not act paternalistically. I accept that paternalism may be

[18]   Other advocates of this view are Chin (2002), and less obviously so, Kultgen (2014).

[19]   In addition, sexist, racist, or similar biases can influence physicians' judgment about what is in their patients' best interests, which also makes paternalism threatening to patients (Quill and Brody 1996, 764).

[20]   Alternatively, one could reject the fiduciary model of the patient-physician relationship as some courts have done (Ryman 2017, 31–2), or oppose the idea that this relationship should be non-paternalistic. Ryman has done the latter (2017), although there, she understands "paternalism" more expansively than I do here. Ryman has also come around to the view that Fiduciary Paternalism ought to be rejected; she and I defend this position in depth in McLeod and Ryman (2020).

inevitable in some fiduciary relationships (e.g., in parent–child relationships);[21] it is simply not inevitable in all of them, and is therefore not inherent to relationships of this type. Let me argue for this position first by elaborating on Fiduciary Paternalism, and second by critiquing it using a conception of autonomy according to which having others rely on one's best judgment is compatible with respecting their autonomy.

Why do supporters of Fiduciary Paternalism assume that a fiduciary necessarily acts paternalistically? They must be skeptical that the fiduciary could respect the beneficiary's autonomy while exercising discretionary authority over this person's interests. Alternatively, or in addition, they could doubt whether beneficiaries in general are capable of providing more than mere generic consent for actions that fiduciaries commit on their behalf. To expand on the first worry, respect for beneficiary autonomy would rob fiduciaries of the power over the beneficiaries' interests that is required for them to be fiduciaries. It would not allow fiduciaries to make the "independent and…unreviewable judgment[s]" that are characteristic of the fiduciary role. Rather, it would rather require them to simply do as their beneficiary asks (Markovits 2014, 217). In that case, the fiduciaries could not respect beneficiary autonomy and still be fiduciaries; they *must* act paternalistically.

The second concern arises because of beneficiaries' lack of expert knowledge, which suggests that their authorization or consent for the fiduciary's actions must be merely "generic" (Kultgen 2014, 407). It must be consent, in other words, not for each of their fiduciary's individual actions or decisions (what I'll call "specific consent"), but for the general undertaking by their fiduciary to act in their best interests (i.e., "generic consent"). If beneficiaries always gave specific consent, then there would be no paternalism in fiduciary relationships. But if instead they gave only generic consent, then there would be paternalism; fiduciaries would have to act on their judgment about what is in their beneficiaries' best interests and without the beneficiaries' informed consent for their individual actions.

In critiquing Fiduciary Paternalism, I want to show how fiduciaries could respect beneficiary autonomy—and therefore obtain specific consent—while at the same time exercising discretionary authority over beneficiaries' interests. Let me begin by explaining how fiduciaries could acquire more

---

[21] As I have argued, fiduciaries are duty-bound to be loyal to beneficiaries' interests. Often this will involve pursuing ends that the beneficiaries set for themselves, although it can entail (i.e., where the beneficiaries are not autonomous), setting ends for them. Where it does so, the fiduciaries must act paternalistically.

than generic consent for their actions despite the knowledge gap between them and their beneficiaries. There are certainly models of informed consent in bioethics that describe how this could happen. Bioethicists stress that physicians need to inform patients about their health care situation in a way that they will understand and help them, if necessary, to interpret relevant information and connect it their values so that they can decide based on them. It can also be appropriate for physicians to make recommendations to patients that are grounded in what physicians know their patient's values to be or even in health-related values that physicians believe their patients should endorse. That is true, at least, so long as the patients feel that they can refuse these recommendations (Emanuel and Emanuel 1992). Physicians need to engage at most in persuasion with patients, and avoid coercion and manipulation, which is admittedly difficult given the power differential between them and their patients. Success in this informed choice process requires that physicians have enhanced communication skills, including skills at making patients with different social backgrounds comfortable enough that they can raise questions and issue clear refusals if they do not like what their physicians suggest for them.[22]

Advocates of Fiduciary Paternalism might say the following: that the support—or in their words, the *interference*—I have just described from physicians for, or with, patient decision-making is inconsistent with physicians' respecting patient autonomy. But such a complaint makes sense only if "autonomy" means freedom from interference, which it does not for most bioethicists. Instead, they define autonomy in terms of self-governance, which is basically the ability to reflect critically on one's situation in light of one's values and information about one's options, and to decide based on them (see, e.g., Emanuel and Emanuel 1992; Quill and Brody 1996; McCullough and Wear 1985; Sherwin 1998; McLeod 2002). Autonomy, so understood, is consistent with receiving the sort of guidance I have described (i.e., from physicians). Indeed, it usually requires such assistance in health care contexts.[23]

---

[22] See McLeod 2002, including on the use of the term "informed choice" rather than "informed consent" (and here, see also Baylis 1993).

[23] Feminist bioethicists, in particular, emphasize this fact. Many of them argue that autonomy, or self-governance, is "relational" (i.e., socio-politically constituted; e.g., Sherwin 1998; McLeod 2002; Mackenzie and Stoljar 2000). On this view, autonomy admits of degrees and the degree of autonomy that people will reach depends, in part, on how much social support exists for their autonomy and how vulnerable they are to political forces of oppression. For a discussion about respect for relational autonomy in fiduciary relationships, see McLeod and Ryman (2020).

Physicians can therefore respect patient autonomy, despite how little expert knowledge patients normally have about medicine, because they can guide them in making autonomous choices about their health care. But can they respect patient autonomy and still wield discretionary authority over patients' interests, which they must do as fiduciaries? I think the process of informed choice actually *requires* that they exercise such authority; it is not merely consistent with it. For example, to be able to present a patient with a diagnosis, prognosis, or treatment options, physicians must employ their discretion—that is, about what the diagnosis, prognosis, and options are, or should be, given the patient's condition (Ryman 2017). Also, during the informed choice process, they must make discretionary judgments about how to present information in a way that patients will understand, about whether patients do understand in the end what they are choosing, about whether they are choosing freely as opposed to being subject to the will of another including the physician's own will, etcetera. Lastly, physicians must carry out the will of their patients, which is part of respecting their autonomy. Usually, such action is an exercise not in mere authority, but in *discretionary* authority; they must use their discretion in deciding how best to perform procedures such as an abortion or egg retrieval during in vitro fertilization.[24]

If physicians can have the discretionary authority of a fiduciary while respecting patient autonomy, then Fiduciary Paternalism must be false; the fiduciary relationship is not inevitably paternalistic. Fiduciary Paternalism is therefore not a threat to the fiduciary model of the patient–physician relationship.[25]

---

[24] That is true, in part at least, because each patient's physical body is different, which often requires that physicians carry out even routine interventions differently on different patients (Ryman 2017).

[25] One might object to this argument by insisting that physicians who are committed to serving their patients' interests should engage, at the very least, in *nudging* their patients. Nudging involves presenting options in such a way that people are more likely to choose the option one thinks is best, because of cognitive biases they have. An example of such a bias is the herd mentality, which can encourage patients to choose a certain health care option if they are told that most patients in their situation do so (Thaler and Sunstein 2008). Since the original literature on nudging defines it as a form of paternalism (i.e., as "libertarian paternalism"), and nudging by fiduciaries seems appropriate, perhaps Fiduciary Paternalism is correct after all.

Let me respond by saying first that it is questionable whether nudging is indeed a form of paternalism, and if it is not, then the argument I've just outlined does not support Fiduciary Paternalism. There is some debate about whether nudging is paternalistic, given that it may not be inherently manipulative or coercive and therefore may not inhibit autonomy (Quigley 2013; Ploug and Holm 2015; Conly 2013). Consider second that if nudging does count as paternalism because it *is* manipulative or coercive, then it is probably not in beneficiaries' interests for fiduciaries to nudge them. The main interest it would violate is that of being autonomous.

My hope is that this discussion has helped not only to ease the worry posed by Fiduciary Paternalism to the model of physicians as fiduciaries, but also to refine our understanding of the fiduciary relationship. Although fiduciaries do have discretionary authority to set or pursue significant practical interests of beneficiaries, they should not further these interests in a way that conflicts with what competent beneficiaries want for themselves.[26] For otherwise, they will compromise their beneficiaries' interests, including their interest in autonomy. They would even cease, arguably, to act on their beneficiaries' behalf. Let me illustrate this last point by returning to Smith's example of backgammon players, Alberta and Belinda. Imagine that Albert knows Belinda has a special strategy for playing backgammon, one that differs from his own. In acting on her behalf, he should make the move that fits with her strategy, not his (if only because he's likely to mess up her game otherwise). It would still be up to him to decide what the best move is according to this strategy; but overall *it* should guide him in determining what is in Belinda's interests.[27] When we act on behalf of others who are autonomous in the sphere in which we act for them, we must take their values into account. Otherwise, it's not clear that we truly act on *their* behalf. Indeed, if that is what fiduciaries are authorized to do—act on other people's behalf—then they must respect their autonomy.[28]

2.4 Pharmacists (etc.)

Health care professionals other than physicians are thought to have similar ethical obligations as physicians, including the obligation to respect patient autonomy and to give primacy to patients' interests. But are these other professionals fiduciaries, or ought they to be regarded as such? Do they have a professional obligation to be devoted to their patients' interests *because* they are fiduciaries? I want to answer these questions first by focusing on

[26] That is not to say they should heed every request made by competent beneficiaries. Some requests (e.g., for medically unnecessary procedures) are not consistent with fiduciaries promoting the interests of their beneficiaries that they have been authorized to promote, or that they perhaps *could* be authorized to promote while acting in their professional capacity (e.g., as a physician). On this last point about what fiduciaries can be authorized to do, see Section 3.2.

[27] To use a similar example, if my son Abeti asked me to play his turn for him in the game *Ticket to Ride*, then I would feel compelled to adopt his cut-throat (though legitimate!) method of playing this game while acting on his behalf. This idea about autonomy and acting on another's behalf comes from Emma Ryman (personal communication).

[28] As Miller would put it, they need to use their discretionary authority to *pursue* the ends of autonomous individuals, rather than set their ends for them.

pharmacists (as I do in other chapters, esp. Chapter 2), and second by generalizing the comments I make about them to other gatekeeping health care professionals.

Some authors writing on conscientious objection in pharmacy are sympathetic to the idea that pharmacists have distinctly *fiduciary* obligations (e.g., Cantor and Baum 2004, 2009; Wicclair 2006, 242). However, others would claim that pharmacists lack the authority of a fiduciary (i.e., to use their discretion to set or pursue significant practical interests of others). Consider the following from Lewis Wall and Douglas Brown:

> Although acknowledged as experts in the nature and action of drugs, pharmacists do not control the use of prescription medications. Pharmacists exercise only technical supervision over the dispensation of medications that are prescribed by physicians. Because pharmacists can dispense but not prescribe medications, their activities are constrained in major ways by the medical profession. Physicians send their patients to the pharmacy to have prescriptions filled, and they retain responsibility for the care of these patients. They do not transfer their care to the pharmacist. The pharmacists who fill such prescriptions (particularly in the commercial retail setting) typically have only the most cursory knowledge of the clinical circumstances in which any given patient's prescription has been written.   (2006, 1149)

Since they lack knowledge of these clinical circumstances, they must exercise little, if any, discretionary judgment about where patients' interests lie in terms of what medications they receive. Pharmacists cannot be responsible for acting in these interests for this reason, and also because this responsibility remains in physicians' hands. One could argue in this way in favor of the view that pharmacists are decidedly not fiduciaries.[29]

Relying on Wall and Brown's conception of the pharmacist's role would be a mistake, however, because their conception is misleading or is, at best, incomplete. It misses at least two key aspects of this role. First, pharmacists can prescribe some drugs; they do not merely dispense drugs that physicians prescribe. The relevant medications include those that are available without a prescription but are behind the counter, which is true in many countries of the EC levonorgestrel (i.e., Plan B; see Schulz et al. 2016 and

---

[29] Although Wall and Brown would clearly endorse this view, they don't do so explicitly (2006).

Chapter 2, note 59). As the gatekeepers to medications like these, pharmacists are responsible for the care of patients who receive them, which means, at a minimum, that they must dispense them only when they are medically indicated and provide counseling about their proper use and known side effects. With respect to EC, for example, pharmacists must decide whether there are drug interactions or contraindications that are relevant to its use by a particular patient,[30] which in turn requires that they have more than a "cursory knowledge" of the patient's clinical circumstances (FSRH 2017, vii).[31] They also must use their judgment to determine how best to inform the patient about the drug. These points suggest that in contexts like these, pharmacists are indeed fiduciaries.

Second, even where pharmacists dispense drugs that physicians prescribe, they are required to use their discretionary judgment to serve patients' health interests, rather than act like mere technicians, as Wall and Brown suggest (Wicclair 2006, 227). Wall and Brown write that pharmacists are expected not "to fill prescriptions that contain *obvious* dosing errors or that pose a dangerous risk of interacting with other drugs, about which the prescribing physician might not be aware" (2006, 1149; my emphasis). In short, they are responsible for trying to prevent "medicine-related errors" (Wiedenmayer et al. 2006, 6). It will not always be "obvious," however, when these problems arise: that is, when the dosage is wrong or—given the complicated nature of many drug–drug interactions (Tannenbaum and Sheehan 2014; Murphy et al. 2004)—when there is a "dangerous risk" of one occurring. Pharmacists need some "scope for judgment" in identifying and responding to these problems (Miller 2011, 273), which are potentially very serious for patients. They are also very common according to Karin Wiedenmayer and colleagues (writing on behalf of the World Health Organization and the International Pharmaceutical Federation), who say that "more than half of all prescriptions are incorrect" (2006, 3). As well as being responsible for deciding which drugs at which doses best serve their patients' interests, pharmacists need to ensure that patients understand how to take their medications properly, which can require pharmacists to use their discretionary judgment. This role of managing patients' drug therapy may be one that pharmacists share to

---

[30] To give an example of a relevant drug interaction, using enzyme-inducing drugs can reduce the effectiveness of EC levonorgestrel (FSRH 2017).

[31] See Rafie et al. (2017) on the role of the "community pharmacist" in delivering EC where pharmacists are the gatekeepers to it.

some extent with physicians, but they have it nonetheless.[32] And if that is true, then pharmacists are fiduciaries, even when they are "merely" filling prescriptions.

Granted, the above explanations for why pharmacists are fiduciaries may not fit every relationship or interaction that pharmacists have with patients. Some pharmacists do not take seriously the role of "drug therapy manager," for instance, seeing themselves more as just dispensers of medication prescribed by physicians (Wiedenmayer et al. 2006, 4, 7). Such a view is understandable, moreover, given that a "paradigm shift" is only now occurring in pharmacy practice away from the latter conception of the pharmacist role— as dispenser (and compounder)—toward the former conception—as drug therapy manager and, I would add, fiduciary (Wiedenmayer et al. 2006, 4).[33] In addition, some patients do not grant pharmacists the discretionary authority required of a fiduciary. Wall and Brown hint at this second objection when they write that "[c]ustomers who go to a drug store do not expect to have a professional encounter similar to what transpires between physician and patient, priest and congregant, or lawyer and clients" (2006, 1149). That is not true of all "customers" of pharmacies (Austin et al. 2006), although it is undoubtedly true of some of them. Pharmacists can, and arguably should, work to change these expectations, especially when they are prescribing drugs for patients. Ultimately, they do need to be authorized by (competent) patients to be their fiduciaries. Where they do not have this authorization or do not themselves engage with patients as a fiduciary would, then they lack this status.[34]

Moving forward, I'm interested in relationships that pharmacists—and other gatekeepers to reproductive services—have in which they do act as fiduciaries. I assume that at a minimum, these interactions include those in which health care professionals decide on their own what would serve the health interests of patients; they do not simply act on the instructions of other health care professionals. These are cases, for pharmacists, where they prescribe medications, which they often do with EC, and for midwives and nurse practitioners, where they decide on and perform procedures

---

[32] Wiedenmayer and colleagues define the pharmacist role as that of "drug therapy manager," rather than mere dispenser and compounder of drugs, a definition that fits with the description I'm offering here (2006, 4). See their work for more details about this role.

[33] The movement favors what has been called "pharmaceutical care," where "all practitioners…assume responsibility [collaboratively] for the outcomes of drug therapy in their patients" (Wiedenmayer et al. 2006, 7). In this model, pharmacists have the kind of direct responsibility for patient care that physicians have (i.e., as fiduciaries).

[34] And here, the "patients" may be better described as "clients" or "customers."

themselves, which they sometimes do with abortions. It is quite clear that while performing these tasks, health care professionals are fiduciaries and therefore have fiduciary obligations including that of loyalty. They may, in other circumstances, take on a different role, including that of a competent technician, where they exercise little to no discretion over patient care.[35] The suggestion that health care professionals other than physicians (e.g., pharmacists or nurse practitioners) are only ever mere technicians is false, however, for they often do have the discretionary authority that is characteristic of fiduciaries.

3. The Fiduciary Model and Conscientious Refusals

Turning finally to the issue of conscientious refusals, what do my claims about health care professionals being fiduciaries suggest about them? I have maintained that physicians are fiduciaries and that other health care professionals, such as pharmacists, are fiduciaries at least while serving in a gatekeeping capacity. I now want to discuss how being a fiduciary might morally restrict one's ability to make conscientious refusals. This matter is obviously relevant for health care professionals only when they assume a fiduciary role. When, or if, they act as mere technicians—as "technical sales clerk[s]," as Robert Veatch has put it (1999, cited in Wicclair 2006, 227)—they should have no more freedom of conscience than anyone else in such a position (which I assume is little freedom of conscience at all).

As I mentioned in the Introduction, the scope of my discussion about conscientious refusals in this chapter is somewhat limited. First, it centers on encounters between patients and objectors who are in an existing (fiduciary) relationship. As I maintain in Chapter 6, these relationships begin when the health care professional first intervenes to serve the patient's health care needs. Second, my discussion here will focus primarily on typical refusals in reproductive health care, which again target services that are standard (legal and professionally accepted) and that the objectors believe will result in the death of a human being that has the moral or religious status of a person (e.g., a fetus or embryo). The objectors often view this "person" as a second patient. Also, because of the nature of their refusals, they may decline not

---

[35] In the legal literature on fiduciaries, there is support for the idea that people can step in and out of the fiduciary role, even in the same relationship. See, e.g., Miller (2014).

only to perform the offending service themselves, but also to make a referral for it to a colleague who is willing or able to provide it, or indeed to offer any useful information about it. My goal here is to defend my prioritizing approach to these refusals using the fiduciary model along with other insights about conscientious refusals, including those about the harm they can cause to patients (as discussed in Chapters 2 and 3) and those that Kolers brings to the debate about support for the aims of the medical profession. As noted above, I will also discuss atypical refusals, though only at the end.

Let me consider two possible scenarios involving typical refusals (i.e., within relationships that are fiduciary). In Scenario 1, the objector wants only to protect her interest in leading a certain moral life, and not to frustrate her patients' interests or indeed to promote them on the grounds that being *denied* access to the requested service is in patients' interests, which is something the objector could insist on. She, the objector, may believe that this is where patients' interests lie; still, she does not refuse patients' requests on these grounds, because she does not feel that her personal moral beliefs should influence her clinical practice to this degree. (At the same time, she might advocate outside of her practice for relevant changes to health policy.)[36]

By contrast, in Scenario 2, the objector is concerned with the interests of his patients, among which he includes fetuses and embryos. The objector makes it clear that he believes the best interests of his patients—of fetuses or embryos at least—require that he not offer reproductive services like abortions. To illustrate, he might tell a patient who requests an abortion that abortion is a sin, which suggests in so many words that the patient's best interests and those of the fetus lie in the request being denied and in the pregnancy continuing. Such an objector clearly aims to promote more than just a personal interest in leading an authentic moral life; he also wants to further an interest he presumes everyone has in saving unborn lives.

In what follows, I aim to give a fiduciary analysis of the objectors' behavior in Scenarios 1 and 2. My ultimate goal, again, is to defend the prioritizing approach to conscientious refusals.

---

[36] Although this is not the place to assess the moral integrity of objectors, let me say briefly that in Scenario 1, the objector's actions in support of her moral beliefs have personal and social value, which means that she could possess moral integrity as I have understood that quality (see Chapter 1). The same is true of the objector in Scenario 2, although his moral integrity could be compromised if he is trying to *dictate* how someone else should lead her moral life, rather than simply contribute to social debate about what is worth doing, morally speaking.

3.1 Scenario 1

It appears the objector in Scenario 1 believes she has a right to freedom of conscience that she can exercise in her relationships with patients. Interestingly, many bioethicists would agree with her about this right. They would also say in cases like hers that we should find a compromise solution that respects relevant rights or interests of both the objector and the patient. A fiduciary analysis of this scenario would be quite different, however; it would center on whether the objector breaches her duty of loyalty and whether this duty is compatible with health care professionals invoking a right to conscience as she does. Such an approach is preferable, in my view, again because it takes seriously the professional role and duties of objectors and of their power relative to their patients.

The question then is whether the objector in Scenario 1 actually violates her fiduciary duty of loyalty? Recall, this duty requires health care professionals to prioritize their patients' interests above their own interests in the sphere of their patients' health. They also must avoid conflicts of interest in this sphere (or at the very least settle these conflicts in the way that is best for their patients). The objector in Scenario 1 does not place her patient's interests above or even on a par with her personal interest in living a certain moral or religious life. That much is clear. But some would contend that the relevant interests of the patients are not of the right sort. (They are not interests that fall within the sphere in which the objector possesses fiduciary authority.) Others might say that a right of conscience for health care professionals can defeat their duty of loyalty, in which case the objector has done nothing wrong. Let me consider each of these objections in turn.

For there to be a violation of the fiduciary duty of loyalty in Scenario 1, the interests at stake for the patients who request the offending service would have to be interests related to their health or health care. Some would say that the relevant interests are not of this sort: that what the patients would sacrifice if their health care professional were allowed to act on her conscience is mere convenience, particularly if the patients live in an area where there is another such professional nearby who could provide them with the services they seek. If they don't obtain these services from their own health care professional, then, on this view, they are simply inconvenienced. Since an interest in convenience is not a health care interest—surely that much is true—there is no breach of the duty of loyalty in this case.

To counter such an objection, I need to look outside of the literature on fiduciaries to the arguments I made in Chapters 2 and 3 about why typical refusals in reproductive health care are not merely inconvenient but rather harm patients, even when they can get the care they need somewhere else close by. These chapters reveal that often the interests at stake for patients in allowing these refusals include their sense of bodily security, their reproductive autonomy, and/or their trust in health care professions and professionals. The first interest involves patients being secure in knowing that they can control what happens to their bodies and that their society respects this need, which is at risk when health care professionals are permitted to make conscientious refusals. The second interest—in reproductive autonomy—can be at stake with these refusals as well, because patients can feel so humiliated or ashamed when they are conscientiously denied services that they decide to give up on their quest for care. In this way, conscientious refusals can compromise patients' reproductive autonomy. They most likely have this effect, moreover, when patients experience intensely the stigma that surrounds controversial services such as abortions (see Chapters 2 and 3 on this stigma).[37]

The third interest named above is that of trust in the objector's profession and fellow professionals. Damage to patients' trust can occur—alternatively or in addition to having their sense of bodily security and reproductive autonomy threatened—when they are denied a reproductive health service on grounds of conscience. Upon them believing or understanding that the profession allows its members to behave in this way, they can come to question its trustworthiness, along with that of its members (i.e., qua members). Indeed, I think a loss of patient trust is highly likely in these cases. I discussed this problem in Chapter 3 and described the other harms—the loss of security and reproductive autonomy—in Chapter 2.

It follows from these earlier chapters that what at stake for patients in allowing conscientious refusals is not mere inconvenience, but very likely trust in relevant health care professions and very possibly a sense of bodily security and reproductive autonomy. These interests are health care interests in the sense that their protection within health care is crucial to patients

---

[37] This point speaks to patients being vulnerable in a circumstantial way because of oppressive norms when they request these services. Yet one might ask whether, insofar as they are fiduciaries, health care professionals are required to attend to circumstantial vulnerabilities of patients that are brought on by oppressive social structures. To respond to this objection, fiduciaries cannot ignore circumstantial vulnerabilities of their beneficiaries. They usually need to attend to them in deciding how best to serve beneficiaries' interests. This fact is made most clear by acknowledging that illness is a circumstantial vulnerability of patients, which health care professionals obviously cannot overlook.

receiving good, respectful health care.[38] Health care professionals who fail to protect them violate their fiduciary duty of loyalty. The objector in Scenario 1 therefore commits this wrong and does so regardless of whether her patients could easily obtain the relevant services somewhere else.

Let me add that the wrong the objector commits in this scenario involves a misuse of authority: more specifically, the authority to grant patients' access to standard services. Rather than use this authority as it is meant to be used—to promote patients' health care interests—the objector uses it to further her own moral integrity. What is troublesome about this case, therefore—like all other cases of conscientious objection, in my view—is that the objector misuses or abuses her power.

One might accept much of this analysis of Scenario 1, however, except for the part about the objector doing wrong. For one might insist that her behavior is justified by the personal value of her acting on her conscience: in other words, of her leading her life by her own moral lights. According to this view, health care professionals have a right to conscience that trumps fiduciary concerns about loyalty to patients; the fiduciary duty of loyalty is a *prima facie* duty that exists only in the absence of conflict with the professionals' conscience and their desire to live their life in accordance with it.

Let me respond by saying that such a view is simply implausible. Health care professionals cannot be both fiduciaries and in possession of a right to conscience that allows them to ignore the health interests of their patients whenever their conscience demands that they do so. Such a right would effectively allow them to have conflicts of interest (or obligation) that their patients may not consent to, and to behave in the face of these conflicts in a way that is disloyal to patients. The right would therefore be incompatible with the central duty of a fiduciary, which is that of loyalty. In short, health care professionals cannot both be fiduciaries and promote their own interests (moral or otherwise) regardless of whether doing so serves relevant interests of their patients. Since the objector in Scenario 1 behaves in this way, her behavior is indeed wrongful.

To summarize my conclusion about Scenario 1: the objector breaches her fiduciary duty of loyalty, because she inappropriately places her interest in living a certain moral life ahead of the health interests of her patient. At the

---

[38] Patients who do not trust health care professions will be reluctant to seek assistance from health care professionals and/or will have poor encounters with them, as will patients who feel that they lack bodily security in such contexts. In addition, patients who are not able to exercise their reproductive autonomy in their interactions with health care professionals clearly do not receive adequate reproductive health care.

very least, she should have provided the patient with a proper referral (i.e., a referral to a colleague who is willing and able to offer the requested service). In fact, given the conflict her conscientious objection created for her as a health care professional, she may have been obligated to make a referral rather than provide the service herself. The fiduciary model allows us to support the referral requirement, for some objectors at least, though not by arguing that a referral amounts to a true or a good compromise (see Chapter 4). Instead, a referral would be justified where the objectors know that in performing the offending service, they cannot be as loyal to their patients as they should be as their fiduciaries. To be clear, objectors' capacity for loyalty should probably be limited in this respect only when they find the relevant service abhorrent, as many typical objectors do of the services that offend them.[39] In all other cases, they should, as professionals, be able to exercise some professional distance and provide the service themselves and do it well (e.g., compassionately) if it is a standard part of a practice like theirs.[40]

3.2 Scenario 2

While the objector in Scenario 1 prioritizes her own interests over those of her patient, the objector in Scenario 2 assumes there is an alignment between his interests and those of his patients, of which there are two in his mind: the person requesting care and a fetus or embryo.[41] The objector comes to this conclusion, moreover, by interpreting his patients' interests using his conscience. The fiduciary model has us question whether health care professionals who behave in this way act outside, or in abuse, of their discretionary authority. Are they authorized normally to appeal to their conscience alone and ignore what is standard of care when deciding whether to accede to patients' requests for this care? No one in the bioethics literature frames the problem in this way, but doing so can be illuminating.

In terms of who or what authorizes health care professionals to intervene on behalf of patients, I have already suggested that it is the patients themselves when they are competent. (The state also plays a role in licensing these professionals to engage in the regulated activities that form their practice, although it is patients—again when they are competent—who authorize the

---

[39] I owe this point to Mianna Lotz (personal communication).
[40] "Professional distance is selectively withholding expression of personal values in professional life" (Martin 2000, 84).
[41] For simplicity, I'll assume we're only dealing with one fetus or embryo.

professionals to intervene for the sake of their health specifically.) For patients who are not competent, the authorization for someone to act on their behalf, such as a family member or a health care professional, comes from law or the state itself via legislation.[42] It follows that if there really are two patients in Scenario 2—the person requesting care and the fetus or embryo—then the objector would have to be authorized by the first patient to appeal only to his conscience in deciding what is best for her (assuming she is competent), and by her or law or the state to decide in this way on behalf of her fetus or embryo.[43]

Focusing first on the competent patient: if she is anything like most patients, then I assume she has not consented to her health care professional acting on his conscience alone, or to ignoring what is standard practice in his profession when those standards violate his conscience. Most patients authorize health care professionals to make decisions on their behalf using not their personal moral beliefs, but rather their professional skill and knowledge. They also expect these professionals to be guided in these decisions by the norms of their profession. I suggested in Chapter 3 that insofar as patients trust health care professionals, they do so in part because of these norms, which give them some sense of what it will mean for them to trust them. Patients don't trust that health care professionals will act on whatever personal beliefs they happen to have, and so do not authorize them to do so either. (Nor, I might add, would it be wise for them to do so if they are marginalized relative to most health care professionals by virtue of their race, sexuality, gender, class, or the like. Their health care professionals' personal morality could be oppressive to them, or their personal experience could be seriously limited in terms of their ability to know what is best for them.)

Not only do most patients not authorize health care professionals essentially to be conscientious objectors, it is not clear that they could do so and still be relating to them as a health care professional. Consider cases that involve patients who attend religiously specialized health care clinics. An example is the pro-life Tepeyac Family Center (now Tepeyac OB/GYN) in Fairfax, VA, whose mission is to "convey the healing presence of Christ through excellent medical care" (as quoted in Lynch 2008, 96; see also Chapter 3). One might think that in such cases, the patients give their health

[42] An example is the *Ontario Health Care Consent Act* (https://www.ontario.ca/laws/statute/96h02; Miller, personal communication).
[43] For simplicity, I use the pronouns "her" and "she" just in this example. Throughout the book, I do not presume that the patients I'm concerned with use these pronouns or have the social identity of a woman. See the Introduction.

care professionals the authority to invoke their conscience, and *only* their conscience, in deciding various dimensions of their care. On the contrary, I think that health care professionals can never really have such authority, not as health care professionals anyway.[44] There are limits to what patients can authorize health care professionals to do *as* health care professionals, and the reason has to do with the social role of these professionals, the aims of their profession, and the need for individual members to be focused on those aims. Such an argument takes us beyond the fiduciary model to the sorts of insights Kolers has about conscientious refusals (2014).

The objector in Scenario 2 therefore acts outside of the authority that his competent patient places, or could legitimately place, in him as a health care professional, when he decides what is in her best interests based solely on his personal conscience. In general, health care professionals do not, and cannot, have such authority over their patients. They are not permitted to act purely in accordance with their conscience, regardless of whether it conflicts with what their patients want or what their profession deems to be the standard of care.

My claim that health care professionals cannot be authorized to act on conscience alone, qua health care professional, is relevant to whether the objector in Scenario 2 could be authorized to behave in this way on behalf of a fetus or embryo. He could not have this authority while inhabiting the role of a health care professional. At the same time, it's not clear how he could obtain the authority to act solely in the interests of the fetus or embryo. His competent patient would not have given him this power surely. The law or the state would not have conferred it on him either, since it permits the service that the objector refuses to provide. (The service must be legal if he is, in fact, engaging in a conscientious refusal; see the Introduction.) Allowing patients to acquire this service (e.g., abortion) is simply not compatible with authorizing health care professionals to protect the lives of fetuses or embryos that are put at risk when patients ask for it.[45] Thus, the objector in Scenario 2 must be acting outside of his authority when he refuses the patient's request because his conscience tells him that doing so best serves the interests of a fetus or embryo.

---

[44] Emma Ryman agrees; this point came from her initially (in personal communication).

[45] There is an additional question here of whether health care professionals could be fiduciaries to fetuses or embryos. Could one have a fiduciary relationship with such an entity, especially an embryo? For relevant discussion, see Ryman (2017, Ch. 4). On the question of whether it would be desirable, as opposed to merely possible, for physicians to occupy this role and perceive these beings as their patients, see Ryman (2017) and Lyerly et al. (2008).

Assuming that typical refusals in reproductive health care are like either Scenario 1 or 2, these refusals are therefore morally problematic. The reasons, in sum, are that the objectors do not prioritize their patients' interests above their own as a loyal fiduciary would, or they prioritize these interests but do not understand them in accordance with the authority that patients or the state have given to them. A further reason, which concerns both scenarios, is that the objectors ignore the autonomous wishes of their patients to receive a standard service, one that is medically indicated in their circumstances. As I said earlier, fiduciaries must respect the autonomy of competent beneficiaries.

3.3 Atypical Refusals

One might accept all that I've said about typical conscientious refusals, but wonder about atypical ones, especially those that are motivated by anti-oppressive values. I gave an example above involving refusals to perform sex-selective abortions of female fetuses. Like the typical refusals in Scenarios 1 and 2, these ones target requests by patients for a service that objectors find morally offensive. I believe that my fiduciary analysis would have us bite the bullet here and insist that objectors in such cases are not authorized—by their patient or anyone else—to use their conscience alone to decide whether their patients will have access to the relevant service. Therefore, they should not block access to it on grounds of conscience or have such action protected by law or by their professional association. That said, the objectors could— and if they want to preserve their moral integrity, they *should* in my opinion— work outside of the clinical setting to change professional norms that are corrupt from their perspective, a move that is open, of course, to all conscientious objectors in health care. This solution, to what is indeed a difficult problem, seems perfectly reasonable to me.[46]

---

[46] Consider that health care professionals could refuse to accede to requests for services like sex-selective abortions on grounds other than conscience. For example, they could insist that the interest some patients have (or claim to have) in bearing male children is not itself a health interest. Moreover, since these professionals are obligated as fiduciaries and as health care professionals to be devoted only to such interests, they should not have to honor these requests. Whether such an argument will succeed will depend on what's at stake for the patients in question (i.e., whether they might face a dire threat to their health if they do not produce a male child. How we understand "health" may also be relevant here; see, e.g., McLeod 2017.) Regardless, the refusal would stem not from personal conscience but from the professionals' understanding of their professional role. It would therefore not be governed by policies on conscientious refusals.

What about conscientious refusals where the patient does authorize the objector's conduct, or, in other words, agrees with the refusal? For the most part, I've used the term "conscientious refusal" to refer to cases where the refusal targets a request by a patient for a particular service, as well as an expectation that the objector will offer this service. At the same time, I acknowledged in the Introduction that "conscientious refusal" can have a wider relevance; it can refer to cases where the target just is the expectation that the objector will provide a certain service (e.g., certain kinds of counseling for abortion), which the patient does not request. Rather, the patient tends to agree that the objector should not offer the service. The example I gave was of a refusal by physicians in the United States to comply with Women's Right To Know (WRTK) laws, which give patients seeking an abortion the legal right to know, and health care professionals the legal obligation to provide, information that is (arguably) unnecessary for, or worse, interferes with, a patient's informed choice in favor of an abortion. I assume that physicians conscientiously objecting to these laws would do so with the implied or express consent of their patients. Their refusals would therefore be atypical, since they would occur *with* the patient's authorization.[47] Let me consider briefly what my fiduciary framework suggests about them.

The refusals themselves appear to conform to the objectors' fiduciary duty to their patients. The objectors exercise discretionary authority rather mere power to do what they judge to be in their patients' health interests. All the while, they prioritize these interests over other interests, including their own and those of public officials who are keen to enforce WRTK laws. Although objectors in these cases may not be morally *required* to subordinate their interests to those of their patients, if only because they wouldn't be much use to their patients if they lost their license (or worse) as a result of breaking the law, they are surely morally permitted to do so. One could apply the fiduciary framework in this way to yield the conclusion that conscientious refusals of this sort are morally permissible.

This conclusion may be too quick, however. Recall the claim I made earlier that patients cannot authorize physicians to use their conscience, and only their conscience, in deciding how to care for them. For they would not be relating to them as physicians if they did that: in other words, if they had no interest in receiving the kind of care that physicians, qua physicians,

---

[47] As I explained in the Introduction, this feature is also present in forms of conscientious conduct other than conscientious refusal, such as conscientious commitment (i.e., action in accordance with a commitment *to provide* services: non-standard ones). I would analyze this conduct similarly to the way I go on to analyze the atypical refusals I've just described.

provide. Although this concern is not a particularly fiduciary one—it has to do ultimately with the integrity of the profession—it is part of my fiduciary analysis of conscientious refusals. It is also important because it allows me to resist the problematic claim that health care professionals, as professionals, are permitted to do *whatever* their patients authorize them to do: that is, to engage in any conduct so long as their patients endorse it.

To show, using the framework I've developed, that objectors who refuse to abide by WRTK laws act permissibly as physicians, I need to demonstrate that their conduct is compatible with the role of a physician, which I believe I can do quite easily. Physicians are obligated to respect their patients' autonomy, which requires that they not provide information about unwanted pregnancies that can mislead patients or that is irrelevant to their abortion decisions. Physicians who oppose WRTK laws understand this very well.

Let me complicate matters further, however, by pointing to circumstances where the dominant conception of the health care professional's role is corrupt—requiring, for example, that these professionals impose treatment on competent patients against their will.[48] Am I not committed to saying that in such circumstances, conscientious refusals that patients authorize and that are motivated by anti-oppressive values are morally *impermissible*? To respond, I would say the opposite on the grounds that there is little moral value in preserving the professional's role so understood and the integrity of the profession that is built around it. At the same time, there *is* moral value in allowing these professionals to use their discretionary *authority* and expertise to decide what they will not do for—or more accurately, *to*—patients. Assuming that these points are correct, the refusals at issue here are morally permissible.

This discussion about atypical refusals has focused on refusals that are prompted by anti-oppressive values. I've had to bite the bullet on some of these cases, but not all of them, by saying that the refusals are morally problematic. They are problematic, in short, when the objectors lack the authority to refuse because their patients disagree with their conscientious conduct. When objectors have this authority, or the blessing of their patients to refuse, the moral circumstances are very different, however; in all likelihood, the refusals are morally permissible.

---

[48] That was the case in Nazi Germany, where some physicians were expected to conduct involuntary experiments on Jewish prisoners. This example comes from an anonymous reviewer of OUP.

I've reserved the term "conscientious refusal" mainly for conduct that pits objectors and (competent) patients against one another. I argued in Section 3 that health care professionals should not be permitted to engage in such behavior because they lack the authority—in other words, the standing—to do so. That is true when there is a fiduciary relationship between them and the patients who make the requests they deny. As fiduciaries, they have discretionary authority to act on their patients' behalves, but they do not have so much discretion that they can appeal to their conscience alone when deciding how to treat their patients. This point applies to typical and atypical refusals (those that generate a conflict with a patient) and is therefore relevant to any general policy on conscientious refusals. Overall, such a policy should not condone this sort of conduct within existing fiduciary patient–health care professional relationships.[49] That said, it could recommend that professionals in these relationships who have conscientious objections make proper referrals for the services that morally offend them when their patients would be better served by someone who doesn't take such offense. Referrals made for the sake not of compromise (see Chapter 4), but of promoting patients' interests cohere with the fiduciary duty of health care professionals to be loyal to their patients.

4. Conclusion

In this chapter, I have defended the prioritizing approach to regulating conscientious refusals made by health care professionals who act as fiduciaries for their patients, which includes all professionals who are charged with playing a gatekeeping role. This approach requires that objectors prioritize their patient's interests over their own personal interests or other interests that support them acting with moral integrity. This demand, in turn, arises from objectors' fiduciary role and from the duty of loyalty that accompanies it. My focus has been mostly on typical refusals and on refusals that occur inside an established, fiduciary patient–health care professional relationship. Whether objectors make their objections inside or outside of such a relationship makes a moral difference, in my view. Chapter 6 examines objections that occur outside of this context.

---

[49] There should perhaps be separate and more permissive policies for atypical refusals that do not create a conflict with a patient, like refusals to abide by WRTK laws. I don't hold out much hope that such policies would be put into place, however, because the relevant behavior must be illegal.

6

Fidelity to Purposes

Most bioethical work on conscientious refusals seeks to answer the general question of whether health care professionals should be free to make these refusals (i.e., free with impunity or without having to justify their actions). From my perspective, this question is too general, however. For me, the context in which health care professionals make their refusals matters morally. What matters, in particular, is whether the refusals occur inside or outside of a fiduciary relationship with a patient. Chapter 5 gave some indication of why I take this stance. There, I argued that health care professionals who have conscientious objections must prioritize patients' interests over their own interest in adhering to their conscience whenever a fiduciary relationship exists between them and their patients. I also clarified that health care professionals tend to have this sort of relationship with patients when they've been tasked with deciding who should receive health care services: in other words, when they are the gatekeepers of health care. The health care professionals I am concerned with throughout this book are professionals of this sort (and so I use the term "health care professional" to refer narrowly to them).

The argument from Chapter 5 applies to objections that health care professionals make to requests for standard services by (or on behalf of) their current patients. It does not concern conscientious refusals that target requests by (or on behalf of) *prospective patients*: that is, people who are not yet the objector's patient but who wish to receive from the objector a standard service that the objector finds morally offensive. The ethics of conscientiously denying standard services to prospective patients as opposed to current ones are distinct, or so I will argue. Much of this chapter centers on this issue, and more precisely on the question, *how free should health care professionals be to refuse to take on new patients because of their conscientious objections?*

My primary objective in this chapter to decide what a general policy on conscientious refusals should say, ethically, about the freedom to take on new patients. Thus, my concern is with all such refusals, not just with those that are typical in reproductive health care. Still, I use examples that involve

Conscience in Reproductive Health Care: Prioritizing Patient Interests. Carolyn McLeod, Oxford University Press (2020).
© Carolyn McLeod.
DOI: 10.1093/oso/9780198732723.001.0001

typical refusals as I did in previous chapters. The question that motivates this chapter is highly relevant to typical refusals, many of which occur outside of a fiduciary relationship with a patient and in, for example, walk-in clinics, emergency rooms, or pharmacies in town or cities where the patient is only visiting. Many patients seek out contraception and abortions from health care professionals who are not their own, which makes the ethics of conscientiously denying requests by prospective patients—and thus refusing to accept them as patients—central to this book.

This chapter has two main sections. Section 1 situates the freedom to choose whether to accept new patients (or which patients to accept) in relation to a freedom that I mentioned in Chapter 2—the freedom "to choose whom to serve" (AMA 2016)—and more generally, to other freedoms that I believe an adequate theory of conscientious refusals in health care should discuss. I clarify my position on these additional freedoms and defend in broad terms my contextualist moral view on conscientious refusals.[1] In doing so, I fulfill a secondary objective of this chapter, which is to give a general summary of my views on these refusals.

Section 2 answers the question in italics above—about the freedom to take on new patients—by appealing to the legal literature on fiduciaries. It is reminiscent in this way of Chapter 5. I argue that health care professionals (again, gatekeepers to health care services) have a duty to the public to promote public health and equitable access to care. What is more, this duty is fiduciary,[2] although it is unique compared to the fiduciary duties that health care professionals have (or can have) toward their individual patients.[3] The duty arises out of a fiduciary relationship that is itself unique in requiring fidelity to certain purposes rather than to a certain individual (or group) (Miller and Gold 2015).[4] The view I defend, in short, is that health care professionals owe their fidelity to the purposes of fostering public health and equitable access to care, and that this requirement restricts their freedom to decline to take on new patients on grounds of conscience. They must

[1] To be clear, my view is contextualist because it insists that the context in which conscientious refusals occur matters, morally speaking.

[2] As in Chapter 5, I am here primarily interested in the moral dimensions of a health care professional's fiduciary role, not its legal dimensions.

[3] I argued in Chapter 5 that for health care professionals other than physicians, their relationships with patients can be, but are not necessarily, fiduciary in nature. These relationships take on a fiduciary character when these professionals act as gatekeepers to reproductive services.

[4] Note that ordinary fiduciary relationships can exist between a person (the fiduciary) and a group, rather than a single individual. An example is a fiduciary who serves the group of all current subscribers to a pension fund (Miller and Gold 2015, 543).

prioritize these purposes over their interest in adhering to their conscience, at least while inhabiting the role as the public's fiduciary. A kind of prioritizing approach is therefore appropriate, in my view, for conscientious refusals that occur outside of established relationships with patients. I conclude that a prioritizing approach that demands fidelity to the purposes I've named should inform general policies on conscientious refusals by health care professionals.

1. Conscience-based Freedoms in Health Care

There are different freedoms health care professionals could have that concern their relationships with patients. These include the freedom to decide *how to serve* their current patients as well as the freedom to choose *whom to serve*, including whether to begin new relationships with patients. Health care professionals could insist on these freedoms for different reasons, including mere preference, conscience, professional obligation, or some combination of all three. To illustrate, physicians might refuse to accede to requests for abortions, because they would simply prefer not to perform abortions given that they find them medically uninteresting. Or physicians might resist forces outside of their profession—such as a government requirement to rein in health care spending—that prevent them from caring well for their patients, and do so on grounds of both conscience and professional obligation. (The two reasons line up with one another in this case; the urge to resist comes from both the physicians' conscience and their sense of professional obligation.) I am interested here in freedoms that pertain to relationships with patients—the formation, continuation, and dissolution of these relationships—that health care professionals exercise for reasons of just conscience. For want of a better term, I call these "conscience-based freedoms."

Two points about conscience-based freedoms are worth making before turning to specific examples. First, these freedoms focus on how health care professionals conduct themselves with current or prospective patients and are therefore relevant to the clinical setting. They do not concern other arenas in which health care professionals might voice their moral objections. As I suggested in earlier chapters, health care professionals do have outlets for their conscience other than the clinic, such as professional meetings, the media, and the blogosphere. Their freedom of conscience therefore extends beyond the clinic and beyond the conscience-based freedoms that

I discuss in this chapter. To restrict these freedoms is not to restrict all freedom of conscience for health care professionals. It may be that limiting their freedom of conscience outside of the clinical setting is appropriate, however; perhaps they would violate a fiduciary duty to the public if they publicly advocated, *as a health care professional,* for a private health care system or for changes to the standards of care of their profession that would diminish the public's access to quality health care. They may need to step outside of their role as a health care professional when voicing these objections.[5] Such limitations on the conscience of health care professionals are not my main focus, although I accept that they may be appropriate, and the position I defend has implications for what they should be exactly.

Second, in questioning the extent to which health care professionals should have conscience-based freedoms, I am interested in whether law or policy should guarantee some accommodation for conscientious refusals.[6] If the answer is no, then these professionals would still be free, of course, to issue their refusals; it's just that they would have to be answerable for them. In that case, their actions would be akin to civil disobedience—that is, "conscientious law-breaking" (that is public and nonviolent; Coady 2016, 501; Rawls 1971; Brownlee 2013; see Chapter 1)—which some argue is a better model for conscientious refusal in health care anyway. For instance, Jeanette Kennett writes that if a "service refusal is indeed a matter of conscience, then the practitioner must be prepared to stand behind this refusal and answer for it" (2017, 78; see also Brownlee 2013).

The nature of what I'm calling "conscience-based freedoms" and the scope of my discussion of them should now be clear. Let me turn to specific examples of these freedoms and to my views on policies about them and conscientious refusals. Parts of this discussion will serve as a review of what I argued for in Chapter 5, which concerned the freedom to choose how to serve one's own patients (i.e., while in a fiduciary relationship with them). Other parts will apply the theory of fiduciary relationships I outlined in that

---

[5] Immanuel Kant deals with this sort of issue in "What Is Enlightenment?" (1784/1996). He argues that people's conscience should be entirely free when they act as "*scholar*[s] before the entire public of the *world of readers,*" but their conscience should be restricted when they assume a "*civil* post or office with which [they are] entrusted" (8:37; his emphasis). In addition, he says that one doesn't violate duties associated with one's post or office if, as a "scholar," one publicly criticizes them. I owe these points to Dennis Klimchuk (personal communication).

[6] Relevant to these freedoms—in particular, the freedom to choose *how to serve*—are forms of conscientious conduct other than conscientious refusals, including conscientious compliance and conscientious commitment (see the Introduction). But I'm interested only in how, or whether, these freedoms should be restricted in ways that inhibit health care professionals from making conscientious *refusals.*

chapter to aspects of the freedom to choose whom to serve. While clarifying my position on different conscience-based freedoms, I will also contrast it with common policies about them, but will omit policies that are uncontroversial. The latter include guidelines stating that health care professionals should not make conscientious refusals in emergencies, or in a way that amounts to invidious discrimination or that interferes with their duty to disclose information about patients' health care options.[7]

1.1 Freedom to Choose How to Serve

One example of a conscience-based freedom is the freedom of health care professionals to let conscience guide their decisions about how to serve their current patients (i.e., people they have already agreed to serve; those with whom they are in an established relationship). In Chapter 5, I suggested that this freedom should not be so extensive that it allows for conscientious refusals. Moreover, to defend this view, I pointed to the (normatively) fiduciary nature of the relationships that exists between health care professionals and their patients (when the former act as gatekeepers in particular).[8] Health care professionals are fiduciaries when they have "standing (authority) to make discretionary decisions for or on behalf of" patients (Miller and Gold 2015, 540). Such authority is never unlimited; importantly, qua fiduciary, health care professionals lack the standing to interpret their patients' interests through the lens of conscience alone when their conscience conflicts with standard practice. This fact does not preclude them, however, from making referrals for a service that they conscientiously object to, rather than offering this service themselves. Indeed, a referral would be obligatory if they knew they could not provide the compassionate care that their patients need because of their conscientious objections. I argued for these claims in Chapter 5.

---

[7] These restrictions are not controversial among bioethicists or among health professional organizations. To give an example involving the latter, the "Ethical Opinions of the Council on Ethical and Judicial Affairs," which is part of the American Medical Association's *Code of Medical Ethics* (2016), says that physicians "have an ethical obligation to provide care in cases of medical emergency," and "may not decline to accept a patient for reasons that would constitute discrimination against a class or category of patients" (AMA 2016, 1.1.2). They also must "inform...patient[s] about all relevant options for treatment, including options to which the physician morally objects" (AMA 2016, 1.1.7).

[8] My claim that these relationships are fiduciary ones was normative; they morally *ought to be* recognized as fiduciary, but may not always be recognized as such.

On the whole, my position on the freedom to "choose how to serve," as I'm calling it, is consistent with policies requiring that health care professionals who conscientiously object to a standard service provide their patients with a proper referral for it.[9] That said, I would recommend rules that are somewhat more stringent than these policies tend to be.[10] Consider that on my account, what is most important about referrals is that they serve patients' interests. That is true because (or when) health care professionals are duty-bound as fiduciaries to prioritize their patients' interests over their own. Thus, referrals should not occur when they are not in patients' interests and a policy on conscientious objection and referral should reflect this fact. Some patients will not want a referral, and for good reason. For example, when the care they need will be emotionally very difficult for them, they might prefer to receive it from a health care professional whom they know and trust even if this person is a conscientious objector. Policies that ultimately force patients to obtain referrals that do not serve their interests are morally unjust.[11]

1.2   Freedom to Choose Whom to Serve

Other conscience-based freedoms concern what the American Medical Association (AMA) calls the freedom "to choose whom to serve" (2016, Principle VI). In electing to serve prospective patients, health care professionals are deciding to form health care relationships with them. That is true according to the widely accepted view that physicians' relationships with patients begin when they first intervene to serve a patient's medical needs (AMA 2016, 1.1.1; Blake 2012, cited in Ryman 2017), a theory that must apply to other health care professionals and their relationships with patients. The freedom to choose whom to serve entails the freedom to choose whether to begin a relationship with a patient, but also whether to end such a relationship. Both concern decisions about whom to serve (or continue to serve).

[9] For an example of a policy requiring that objecting *pharmacists* provide referrals, see the Ontario College of Pharmacists' "Professional Obligations When Declining to Provide a Pharmacy Product or Service due to Conscience or Religion" (2016). I discussed similar policies for physicians in Chapter 4.

[10] That includes the model policy for physicians that I and others have recommended (Downie et al. 2013). According to this statement, physicians can make referrals mainly "to protect their own freedom of conscience" (2013, 31). I now believe that referrals should protect patient interests.

[11] Interestingly, this conclusion follows not just from my prioritizing approach to conscientious refusals, but also from the compromise approach (see Chapter 4). The reason is that referral is not a true compromise for patients if it in no way serves their interests.

The larger freedom—to choose whom to serve—thus includes two smaller freedoms that pertain to whether or when to end a relationship with a patient and whether to begin such a relationship in the first place.

These smaller freedoms can both be conscience-based, that is, deployed on grounds of conscience. For example, after receiving a request for an abortion (or a similar service that destroys or threatens "unborn lives"), anti-abortion physicians might decide that their patient's values do not fit well enough with their own for the relationship to continue. So, they decide to try to end it. It is not enough for them to exercise the freedom to choose *how* to serve the patient, which would involve serving them in the way they see fit. Instead, they want to be free of this relationship altogether.

Health care professionals can also choose based on conscience whether to begin relationships with patients. To illustrate, pharmacists could reject requests for emergency contraception (EC) by prospective patients because they, the pharmacists, find EC morally offensive. In doing so, they are deciding for reasons of conscience not to form a relationship with a patient. As I have explained, such conduct and the freedom it involves (i.e., to choose whether to take on new patients) are the main focus of this chapter. Before turning almost exclusively to it, let me comment further briefly on the freedom to end relationships with patients.

How free should health care professionals be to end their relationships with patients? It is widely accepted within health care ethics that health care professionals have a duty not to abandon their patients, an idea that is reflected in the codes of ethics of many health professional associations.[12] What could explain the duty of non-abandonment, however, and what exactly does it require of health care professionals? Some medical associations go into detail about what they believe it does require. For example, some invoke a rather strict policy stating that a physician who intends to terminate a relationship with a patient must facilitate (or "assist in facilitating") the continued care of the patient by another physician (e.g., Australian Medical Association 2016, 2.1.12). By contrast, other associations say that it

---

[12] Further on, I mention relevant medical association policies. To give an example that involves nurses, the Canadian Nurses Association *Code of Ethics for Registered Nurses*, in a segment on "Ethical Considerations in Addressing Expectations That Are in Conflict with One's Conscience," states that "Nurses may not abandon those in need of nursing care" (CNA 2017, Appendix B). Pharmacy codes of ethics also tend to insist that pharmacists are duty-bound to ensure (or make "reasonable efforts to ensure") continuity of care, which means that they cannot simply abandon their patients (Ontario College of Pharmacists 2015, 2.15; see also Pharmaceutical Society of Australia, Principle 1h, 2017; International Pharmaceutical Federation 2014).

is enough for the physician to give the patient "reasonable notice" of this intention (to use the language of the Canadian Medical Association 2018). To determine which sort of policy is best, morally speaking, we must understand what grounds the duty physicians and other health care professionals have not to abandon their patients, and what restricts their freedom simultaneously to end their relationships with patients.

My fiduciary analysis of conscientious refusals in Chapter 5 has clear implications for this freedom. The fiduciary duty of loyalty of physicians to their patients gives them a duty not to abandon them. Insofar as other health care professionals are fiduciaries for their patients, they have these duties as well. To fulfill the (fiduciary) duty of non-abandonment, health care professionals must do more than provide patients with reasonable notice of their intention to end their relationship with them; for they could easily do this much without protecting—or being loyal to—their patients' interest in continuity of care. Instead, they should facilitate the transfer of patients to a colleague (unless, of course, the patients reject such assistance and insist on finding alternative care on their own). To demand less of health care professionals would be to ignore their fiduciary duty of loyalty to their patients. So that they cohere with this duty, policies on the freedom to terminate relationships with patients should also require those who wish to exercise this freedom to have reason to believe that the relevant (fiduciary) relationships will no longer be effective and that dissolving them therefore serves the patient's interests. In that way, conscience would be available to objectors as an excuse only to end relationships that cause them moral distress so significant that it interferes with their ability to care properly for their patients. The fiduciary model demands this limitation to their freedom of conscience, which I believe is a welcome result. Surely, we do not want health care professionals to be free to end all relationships with patients that cause them some moral discomfort.

More could be said about conscience and the dissolution of relationships with patients (especially given that little is said about this topic in the bioethics literature on conscientious refusals). Yet I want to center my attention on the *formation* of these relationships, and on health care professionals who are reluctant to form them for reasons of conscience. The remainder of this section provides some background to this issue and to Section 2, where I defend my position on the conscience-based freedom to decline to take on new patients.

Assuming, again, that the provision of health care service marks the beginning of a patient–health care professional relationship, health care professionals can exercise the conscience-based freedom to begin new relationships with patients in one of three ways. First, they can receive requests for service from prospective patients or from colleagues who refer new patients to them and deny the requests that do not cohere with their conscience. Second, they or their employers can arrange it so that they do not come in contact with prospective patients who wish to receive services that morally offend them. For instance, Maria Bizecki, a pharmacist in Canada who came under fire for refusing to fill prescriptions for what she viewed as abortifacients, "now works in a store where prescriptions are taken in by a technician and put in a basket. She takes only non-objectionable prescriptions to fill from the basket" (Mastromatteo 2003, quoting Michael Izzotti from Pharmacists for Life International-Canada). Third, health care professionals can publicize their conscientious objections in the hopes of avoiding relationships with patients who will request the services they morally object to. Some objectors in Canada have used this method, particularly those who work at walk-in clinics, with one physician in Calgary posting a sign saying she will not prescribe the birth control pill (Krishnan 2014), and another in Ottawa providing a letter to prospective patients stating that he does not prescribe the morning-after pill "or any artificial contraception," nor does he refer patients for vasectomies or abortions (McLeod 2014).

To elaborate on this third method,[13] it is a common policy to require of physicians in particular that before entering relationships with patients, they give prior notice of conscientious objections to providing services that patients could reasonably expect them to provide (see, e.g., AMA 2016, 1.1.7; Downie et al. 2013, 30). Such a strategy is meant to prevent conflicts of conscience from arising in the first place, although it provides no guarantee against them of course. Despite receiving prior notice of a conscientious objection to abortion, for example, patients who thought they would never request an abortion might do so anyway upon finding themselves in an unwanted pregnancy. They could be among the many patients who identify or once identified as anti-abortion, but who eventually have an abortion (see Chapter 3; Cockrill et al. 2013). Cases like these—where the patients want to obtain a service having been told before their relationship with their health care professional began that this person conscientiously refuses to provide it—are complex. They concern both the freedom of these professionals to choose how to serve (i.e., patients to whom they have given prior notice), and their freedom to choose whom to serve, and whether exercising

---

[13] I discuss the second method further below.

the latter by delivering prior notice of refusals to perform certain services is even ethical knowing that some of one's patients may come to need these services. This practice may indeed be unethical for this reason, among others.[14] But rather than take a firm stand on this issue, let me say simply that where prior notice fails to have the intended effect of allowing health care professionals to avoid conflicts of conscience in their relationships with patients, the same moral rules apply as in cases where objectors do not use this tactic: that is, as fiduciaries (or insofar as they are fiduciaries), the objectors must prioritize the interests of their patients over their own interests in abiding by their conscience, since that is what the fiduciary duty of loyalty demands. The duty exists because of the nature of the relationship between the parties, not because of any sort of agreement between them (see Chapter 5, p. 126). It can therefore require that fiduciaries give primacy to beneficiaries' interests, even in cases where they reveal to their beneficiaries ahead of time that they have interests that might conflict with their beneficiaries' interests (see Chapter 5). Although I say more about prior notice below, my general position on it is that it can't morally protect health care professionals against having to engage in health care practices to which they conscientiously object.

Before concluding this part of the chapter, let me comment briefly on cases where health care professionals refuse to take on new patients who request services that they, the professionals, find morally offensive, because having conscientiously refused to receive training in these services, they are now not competent to provide them. I discussed cases like these—of "deliberate incompetence"—in Chapter 3 and treated them as instances of conscientious refusal. Given what I have said about other conscientious refusals, my position on these refusals should be fairly clear: health care professionals should not be able to use conscience as an excuse not to learn how to provide standard services (e.g., those they are expected to provide given their specialty), since they will be obligated to do so when it is in the interests of patients with whom they have a fiduciary relationship to receive these services from them rather than from a stranger or from no one at all (i.e., in circumstances where they are the only health care professional available to the patient). They will also be required to deliver these services in emergencies.

---

[14] The other reasons include the fact that like any form of conscientious refusal, prior notice can diminish the trust people have in the objector's profession (Chapter 3), or can—in reproductive health care contexts—threaten patients' reproductive autonomy, sense of security, or moral identity (Chapter 2).

To summarize Section 1, I've introduced conscience-based freedoms, which are freedoms health care professionals exercise on grounds of conscience that concern their relationships with patients. They include the freedom to choose how to serve patients with whom health care professionals have an existing relationship, and the freedom to choose whom to serve by deciding whether to end existing relationships or to begin new ones. I suggested at the outset that a theory of conscientious objection should cover each of these freedoms individually, and the reasons for that are threefold. First, the grounds for restricting them may differ, depending on whether the freedom occurs inside or outside an established relationship with a patient, which is the case according to my theory of conscientious refusals. Second, the extensiveness of these freedoms can differ. For example, medical codes of ethics tend to give physicians more freedom outside of patient–physician relationships, where turning down prospective patients is largely permitted,[15] than inside of them, where abandoning patients is strictly prohibited. Third, procedures or policies one will want to recommend with respect to these freedoms will likely differ. For example, one will need to say what health care professionals should do when they face the following sorts of conflicts of conscience: ones that prompt them to want to end a relationship that has become ineffectual versus ones that prevent them only from providing a certain service or providing it well within a relationship that they hope will continue. One's guidance here will vary unless, of course, one insists that health care professionals should never allow their conscience to interfere with their professional practice.

2. Freedom to Take on New Patients

I accept that some freedom to choose whether to begin new relationships with patients is warranted for health care professionals. These professionals

---

[15] Doing so is often permitted for a variety of reasons, and those reasons generally include conscience. See, for example, the guidance offered about prospective patients (1.1.2) in the AMA's "Ethical Opinions of the Council on Ethical and Judicial Affairs." The Canadian Medical Association's *Code of Ethics and Professionalism* states simply that physicians have a "right to refuse to accept a patient for legitimate reasons" (plural), which suggests that multiple reasons count as legitimate (2018, 3). The Australian Code, which is more in keeping with my view about the freedom to take on new patients, adds the restriction that an "alternative health care provider" must be available to the patient for it to be legitimate to decline "to enter into a therapeutic relationship" with the patient (2016, 2.1.11).

cannot be obliged to take "all comers" (Fenton and Lomasky 2005, 581–2),[16] if only because they could become overwhelmed and unable to care properly for the patients they have taken on or they could be required to administer treatment that they deem to be futile. To put the point in terms of the duty to treat, which I discussed in Chapter 2, health care professionals do not have this duty toward, and hence a duty to form a health care relationship with, everyone who requests care from them. In short, since they can have good reasons to decline to enter these relationships, they should have some freedom to decide whether to do so. My question is whether conscience should be recognized as one of these reasons. Should health care professionals be free to refuse to take on new patients because of their conscience? Should they be able to decline all requests, made by or on behalf of prospective patients, for services that morally offend them, and also refuse to provide proper referrals for these services? Health care professionals do not, after all, have a duty of loyalty to *prospective* patients; they need not be devoted to these people's individual interests. What then could constrain their conscience-based freedom to choose whether to form relationships with them? My answer, in brief, is a fiduciary duty of loyalty to the public and to the purposes of promoting public health and equitable access to care.

Consider first that too wide a freedom to turn down prospective patients can interfere with access to care and ultimately with public health, among other values (e.g., public trust in health care professions).[17] If the only limits to this freedom are that health care professionals cannot exercise it in emergencies or in a way that is invidiously discriminatory (see the introduction to Section 1), then in regions where many health care professionals object to a certain service, such as abortion, access to it will be poor. This sort of problem exists in some rural areas, but also in whole countries, including Italy. As Alberto Guibilini writes (in 2014), "69% of Italian gynaecologists conscientiously object to performing abortions; in some areas...the percentage is above 85%. Clearly, this situation significantly impacts the actual opportunities women have to access safe abortion" (Guibilini 2014, 167; see

[16] By this I mean accept into their practice all prospective patients who want to receive care from them. They could be required, when their practice is full, to put all new prospective patients on a waiting list, but doing so is not the same as "taking all comers." The motivation to clarify this point comes from an anonymous reviewer from OUP.

[17] A decline in access to care caused by too much conscientious objection can jeopardize public trust (i.e., the trust that people have qua member of the public rather than qua patient). Much of what I say in Chapter 3 about the damage to trust from conscientious refusals is relevant to understanding this threat.

also Chavkin et al. 2017, 59).[18] It negatively affects not only access but also public health, since poor access to safe abortions is a serious—some say a "staggering"—public health problem (Haddad and Nour 2009; see also Grimes et al. 2006).

Of course, too much conscientious refusal can also restrict access to care *within* patient–health care professional relationships. Patients in Italy who already have a gynecologist are not likely to receive an abortion from their gynecologist, because of the situation Guibilini describes. Too much conscientious refusal is also a barrier to patients receiving care via referrals from their current health care professional(s). Presumably, many family physicians in Italy have no hope of providing proper referrals for abortion to gynecologists for patients who either do not yet have a gynecologist or who have one who conscientiously objects to abortions.

Since it can restrict access to care, therefore, the conscience-based freedom to take on new patients must be limited beyond emergencies and cases where the objector's conscience is sexist, racist, or the like. One might agree with this statement, but also contend that the best way to deal with conflicts of conscience that occur outside of a patient–health care professional relationship is to devise some sort a compromise, one that preserves the objector's conscience to some extent while also furthering relevant interests of the public and the profession. In previous chapters, I argued against a compromise approach to conscientious refusals, however, and did so on two grounds: 1) it will not work, at least not for typical refusals in reproductive health care (Chapter 4); and 2) it ignores the fiduciary nature of the relationships that health care professionals have (or can have) with patients (Chapter 5). Although this second point is not relevant to objections that these professionals make to taking on new patients, the first point may indeed be relevant to them. It applies, for example, to cases where the objections are absolute—the objectors refuse to participate *in any way* with the procedure that offends them (e.g., abortion)—making it unreasonable for them to agree to any sort of compromise. Assuming that is correct, the compromise approach will not work for all conscientious refusals that occur outside of an established relationship. At the same time, health care

---

[18] South Africa is another country in which physician conscientious objection has had this effect (Harries et al. 2014; cited in Fiala and Arthur 2017). As I and Lori Kantymir have written, "too much conscientious objection in some parts of the world has made it impossible for health care professions[,] governments[, or hospitals] to meet their commitments to provide certain kinds of health care, especially abortions" (2013, 18, citing Laurance 2007; see also Meyers and Woods 1996; van Bogaert 2002; Koegh et al. 2019).

professionals might have a duty (or duties) that would make certain kinds of compromises in this context morally inappropriate. I turn to this possibility now.

2.1 A Fiduciary Duty to the Public

In my view, health care professionals have a duty to the public that can require them to prioritize the public's interests in public health and equitable access to care over their own interest in abiding by their conscience. What is more, this duty is a fiduciary one. The claim that these professionals have some sort of obligation to the public or to society is not new; it appears in acts that govern the licensing of many health care professionals and in their professions' codes of ethics. What is new, however—to the bioethics literature at least[19]—is the idea that this obligation is fiduciary in nature. Understanding the duty in this way is accurate and also useful; it allows us to see what the duty requires of health care professionals, and how and why it can restrict their conscience-based freedom to refuse to take on new patients.

Health care professionals are licensed by regulatory boards and granted a monopoly (or near monopoly)[20] over the provision of health care services that they are responsible for administering. They are expected, in turn, to promote certain ends, which typically include, among others (e.g., public safety), public health and access to care. These requirements are made clear in acts that govern the regulation of health care professionals. For example, according to Ontario's Regulated Health Professions Act, the health professions must be "regulated and co-ordinated in the public interest, [and]…individuals [must] have access to services provided by the health professions of their choice" (S.O. 1991 Ch. 18, 3).[21] Furthering the public interest in health (i.e., promoting public health) involves providing access that is at least roughly equitable; the two ends of public health and equitable access to care are clearly linked. The idea that health care profes-

---

[19] It is new to the bioethics literature, although it has been developed somewhat in the legal literature on fiduciaries by Evan Criddle and Evan Fox Decent (2018).

[20] Elizabeth Fenton and Loren Lomasky say with respect to pharmacy that it "is not a monopoly; it is more the nature of a cartel or guild. Drug dispensers do compete with each other on price, service, and amenities. They are, however, shielded from competition by non-pharmacists" (2005, 586). From this, I assume that pharmacy and the like are near monopolies.

[21] An example specific to a particular health care profession is the Model State Pharmacy Act in the United States, which requires that pharmacists act in the interests of public health (National Association of Boards of Pharmacy 2003, cited in Wicclair 2006, 228).

sionals are duty-bound to serve them specifically receives support from their professional associations. For instance, the AMA *Code of Medical Ethics* says that "[p]hysicians...have a long-recognized obligation to patients in general to promote public health and access to care" (2015, 11.1.2).[22] And Principle IX of this code specifies that a "physician shall support access to medical care for all people" (2016). Likewise, within the Australian code for pharmacists is the principle that pharmacists must exercise their "professional judgment...in the interests of the wider community" and "promote...equit-able...use of...healthcare resources" (Pharmaceutical Society of Australia 2017, Principle 3). One can find similar requirements for nurse practitioners and midwives in their professional associations' policies.[23] Promoting the health of "the wider community" and equitable access to care is obviously not something that individual health care professionals can do on their own. They should shoulder this moral burden along with their profession and their colleagues in it.[24] Indeed, I presume that is the case below.

What might a duty to promote public health and equitable access to care require of health care professionals? The answer is: many things. For example, they must "be prudent stewards of the shared societal resources with which they are entrusted" so that as many patients as possible can benefit from these limited resources (AMA 2016, 11.1.2). They also, arguably, should not deny access to care based on the ability to pay (i.e., in a private health care system).[25] In addition, the duty could demand that they not make conscientious refusals that prevent members of the public who are not yet their patients from obtaining the care they need. Most of the associations whose

---

[22] According to the Canadian Medical Association, two of the responsibilities of physicians are to "support the profession's responsibility to act in matters relating to public and population health" and to "promote equitable access to health care resources" (2018; points 39 and 40). The Australian medical code, in turn, states that physicians should "accept a share of the profession's responsibility to society in matters relating to the health and safety of the public..." (2016; 4.3.2), should "endeavor to improve...access to medical services in the community" (4.6.1), and should advocate for the "transparent and equitable allocation" of health care resources (4.4.3).

[23] For example, the Canadian Nurses Association *Code of Ethics* states that nurses should advocate for or promote the accessibility of health care services and should also act "for the benefit of the public" (Part II, "Ethical Endeavours Related to Broad Societal Issues," 2017). In addition, according to "The Canadian Midwifery Model of Care Position Statement" by the Canadian Association of Midwives, which is intended as a reference for midwives, "midwifery services in Canada must be universally accessible to all people wherever they live..." (2015).

[24] Some codes of ethics acknowledge this fact explicitly. See note 22, where I quote from the Australian Medical Association's code, which states that physicians must "accept a share of the profession's responsibility to society" (2016; 4.3.2).

[25] That is an expectation of American physicians (AMA 2016, 11.1.4).

codes I have cited do not restrict conscientious objections in this way (not explicitly),[26] although in my view, they should do so.

In what follows, I will provide a moral grounding for the expectation that regulatory boards and professional associations place on health care professionals to promote public health and access to care. The grounding comes from the fiduciary nature of the relationship these professionals have with the public, particularly when they are acting as gatekeepers of health care services. I will argue that while serving in this capacity, these professionals have a *fiduciary* duty to the public, that the duty demands their loyalty to the purposes of furthering public health and access to care, and that this loyalty must take priority over their conscience though it can leave some room for the expression of their conscience. Two caveats about this discussion are in order. First, when I refer to fiduciary duties or relationships, I assume that they can be understood in a moral or a legal sense. As in Chapter 5, I'm primarily interested in their moral dimensions, although I turn to the legal literature to understand their basic characteristics.

Second, when I mention the "public," I mean the following: the group or collective made up of individuals who live in the jurisdiction where the health care professionals in question are licensed to practice. What makes the public in any jurisdiction a collective is that its members share interests (e.g., medical ones) that they hold jointly, rather than severally (Jones 2016,

---

[26] Consider that among the reasons the AMA gives for why physicians might legitimately refuse to accept a new patient are that the patient's request for care "is incompatible with the physician's deeply held...beliefs" (1.1.2.(a)). For its part, the Australian Medical Association has a position statement on conscientious objection that refers to how such conduct can disrupt "the delivery of health care," but the obligations it gives to physicians to prevent this outcome mainly concern their relationships with existing patients (2013). The only directive it gives that would obviously affect prospective patients is that objectors must provide prior notice of their objections. Similarly, a recent Canadian Medical Association's policy statement on MAID suggests that although conscientious objectors have a duty of non-abandonment to existing patients, they have no obligation towards prospective patients (2017). The statement assigns the duty of access to MAID for prospective patients entirely to "health systems" in Canada: "To enable physicians to adhere to [their] moral commitments without causing undue delay for patients pursuing [MAID], health systems will need to implement an easily accessible mechanism to which patients can have direct access." Lastly, the Pharmaceutical Society of Australia (PSA) requires that pharmacists who conscientiously refuse to honor a patient's request for "certain forms of health care...facilitate...continuity of care for the patient" (2017, Principle 2h). (For a similar statement, see the Canadian Nurses Association *Code of Ethics*, Appendix B, "Ethical Considerations in Addressing Expectations That Are in Conflict with One's Conscience," Appendix B, 2017.) In the PSA statement, "patient" could refer to a current or prospective patient. If it does have this referent, then this association's policy is the strongest of the lot.

1; Raz 1986, cited in Jones).[27] An interest in *equitable* access to care, versus mere access to care, is an interest of this sort. It is held by members of the public qua members of this collective, rather than qua individuals, and it is therefore a collective interest. This interest is also tied to a larger collective interest that people have in public health. Although people have an interest in their own health as individuals, they have an interest in public health only as members of a collective (i.e., the public).

2.1.1 Why fiduciary?

Why think that health care professionals have a duty to the public (so understood) that is fiduciary in nature? Recall the theory of fiduciary relationships from Chapter 5, which I borrowed primarily from Paul Miller (and to a lesser extent from Smith 2014; Miller 2011): a fiduciary relationship is a relationship of power in which one party, the fiduciary, has discretionary authority over significant practical interests of the other, the beneficiary. Moreover, the beneficiary is vulnerable to the fiduciary misusing or abusing this power. Let me demonstrate why this theory applies to health care professionals in their relationship to the public and its access to health care.[28] I will also consider objections to this view, or more specifically, to the attempt to describe the duty these professionals have to the public as a fiduciary duty. While answering these concerns, I will explain how the fiduciary role that health care professionals play in relation to the public, while acting as gatekeepers to health care, is unique compared to the one that they do (or may) inhabit in their relationships with patients.

As I discussed in Chapter 5, fiduciaries are people who possess a distinctive type of power over others: power that is discretionary, that exists in the form of authority rather than mere influence or control, and that is authority over the "significant practical interests" of another. Do individual health care professionals have this sort of power over the public? It is undeniable that they (the health care professionals I'm concerned with) have power over who obtains health care services and when they do so. As well, this power is discretionary, meaning there is "scope for judgment in the exercise of it"

---

[27] I do not assume that the public is a group in the stronger sense of having its own unique identity and moral standing which is not reducible to that of its individual members (see Jones 2016). I sincerely doubt that the term "public," as it is used in this context, could refer to a group of this sort.

[28] I have been inspired in doing so by Emma Ryman's application of this theory to the relationships that physicians have with patients who act as gestational surrogates. See Ryman 2017, Ch. 2.

(Miller 2011, 273). Health care professionals use their judgment and expertise in deciding how they will deliver health care services and whom they will deliver them to (i.e., the services for which they act as gatekeeper). These actions of health care professionals affect not only the individual interests of people in their own health, but also their collective interests in public health and equitable access to care. Thus, health care professionals wield discretionary power over these interests of the public.

But is the discretionary power just described "properly understood as authority" (Ryman 2017, 66)? Consider that fiduciaries don't just have power to use their discretion to influence what happens to beneficiaries, as someone might who stages an intervention in a life of a friend who has an addiction. Instead, they have the *authority* to do so, which I assume the interventionist lacks (i.e., because of the very nature of an intervention in the life of an addict). Indeed, health care professionals have authority rather than mere power over the provision of health care services. Their authority comes from the regulatory boards that license them to perform this task, rather than from the public directly, although in granting health care professionals this power, licensing boards certainly act in the interests of the public, as we have seen.[29] They confer the licenses with the expectation that individual health care professionals will promote public health and access to care, among other interests of the public. It is not uncommon for fiduciaries to have their authority granted to them by people or entities that represent their beneficiaries' interests rather than from the beneficiaries themselves. An example is the legal authority that the law gives to parents, who are the fiduciaries of their children.

In applying the fiduciary framework to health care professionals' relationships to the public, a further question we need to ask is whether the discretionary authority they have over the public is the authority to promote significant practical interests. Being a fiduciary doesn't just involve having discretionary authority, since some people have such power yet are clearly not fiduciaries (e.g., personal trainers). The authority must be to affect someone's significant practical interests, which I defined, following Miller, as interests that one promotes while exercising a legal capacity (Miller 2011, 71). The relevant capacity need not be overtly legal, like the capacity to enter into legally binding contracts, but can include, for example, making "decisions relating to [someone's] health and personal welfare" (Miller 2014, 71; Ryman 2017, 67).

---

[29] One could argue that members of these boards are themselves, therefore, fiduciaries for the public.

Health care professionals do make decisions of this sort for members of the public: for example, in choosing when they will have access to health care services. Moreover, in doing so, they affect the collective interests of the public in public health and equitable access to care.

The public is also vulnerable to health care professionals misusing or abusing their authority over the provision of health care services. Vulnerability of this kind is structural in that it exists because of structural features of the relationship these professionals have with the public, specifically features that concern their power over the public. Health care professionals would misuse or abuse this power if they directed it toward furthering their self-interest or the interests of third parties (e.g., manufacturers of drugs or medical devices), rather than those of the public. Consider an example from Chapter 2 of family physicians who, "out of moral indifference to unhealthy people and out of concern for their own lifestyle...refuse to take on new patients who are unhealthy and whom they feel would take up too much of their time." These physicians basically choose new patients based on whether they, the physicians, perceive them to have complex medical needs. They select the patients who do not have these needs, a practice that some call the "cherry picking" of patients (Milne et al. 2014). Physicians who pick their patients in this way use their power over the provision of medical services not for the purposes for which it was given (e.g., to improve public health) but for the sake of their own comfort.[30] Such action constitutes an abuse, or at the very least a misuse, of power.[31]

Health care professionals therefore have discretionary authority over significant practical interests of the public, and the public is vulnerable to them abusing or misusing this power. All the hallmarks of a fiduciary relationship are present in their relationship with the public, and so this relationship must be fiduciary. Assuming this assessment is correct, health care professionals owe the public a duty of loyalty, which is the central duty of fiduciaries. It exists to protect beneficiaries against the abusive exercise of fiduciary power, and more specifically against exploitation. As I explained in Chapter 5, whenever one has discretionary power over another's interests, there is a

---

[30] The point here is not that concern for one's personal comfort is morally inappropriate in the health care professions, but that it should not drive health care professionals in making decisions about who should have access to medical care. Indeed, they should pay attention to their own happiness, if only because they will be better fiduciaries for their patients and the public as a result.

[31] It threatens the collective interests of the public in equitable access to care and public health. The risk it poses to these interests is especially high, of course, when physicians cherry pick en masse.

chance that one will exploit them, or, in other words, take unfair advantage of their vulnerable state.[32] The need to guard against this risk is what morally grounds the fiduciary duty of loyalty. My view is that health care professionals have this duty not only toward individual patients, but also toward the public, and more specifically to members of it qua members, who are the potential victims of exploitation in this context. This duty of loyalty, in turn, informs the duty they have towards the public to promote equitable access to care and public health.

Let me add that being a fiduciary for, and having a duty of loyalty to, the public is not unusual. Among the many fiduciaries of this sort that appear in the legal literature on fiduciaries are trustees for charitable purpose trusts (where property is held in trust and dedicated to a public purpose such as education) and people who run government or state-owned corporations that serve a public purpose, such as providing transportation or postal services (Miller and Gold 2015, 528–30, 532). My contention is that compared with these individuals or entities, health care professionals are in a similar power relationship with the public because they control public access to health care services.

There are objections, of course, that one could raise to this claim about health care professionals being fiduciaries for the public. Let me consider first objections that I believe merit relatively straightforward responses, before turning to one that requires me to add nuance to my view. The first group of objections includes a concern about conflicts of obligation, which fiduciaries are meant to avoid, as I discussed in Chapter 5. Being loyal to the public specifically by promoting equitable access to care can conflict with being loyal to one's patients, if the former involves taking on more patients than one can handle, thereby compromising the care that one can provide to current patients. Such an outcome is indeed a worry, and yet presumably it will arise only in circumstances where there is a shortage of health care professionals. Consequently, it speaks against not the fiduciary model of the relationship these professionals have with the public, but a health care system that does not make enough of them available to the public. (For a similar response to the same sort of objection, see Chapter 5.) In a well-run system, health care professionals should not frequently—which is not to say

---

[32] The explanation I gave specifically was that the discretion makes it possible for fiduciaries to convince themselves that they are fulfilling their mandate when in fact they are acting selfishly or in the interests of a third party (see, e.g., Miller 2011; Smith 2014). Their discretionary power therefore "entails a risk of biased or corrupted judgment," which is then managed by the duty of loyalty (Miller and Gold 2015, 563).

never—experience conflicts of duty that leave them torn between helping current patients or prospective ones.

A further concern is that the fiduciary role I have described does not exist for health care professionals who work in a private rather than a public health care system, which is the case for health care professionals in the United States for example.[33] One might think that in this sort of context, health care professionals have no duty, fiduciary or otherwise, to the public, since the public does not pay them. Instead, they owe their fidelity only to their HMO (or the like) or to individual patients who pay out of pocket.

In response, I could accept that my argument applies only to health care professionals who work within public health care systems; if that were true, then this chapter would still advance the debate on conscientious refusals (particularly refusals made by health care professionals who work within these systems). However, I don't see why I should accept that, because regardless of how health care professionals get paid, they alone are licensed to offer their health care services to the public, and consequently are in the sort of relationship with the public that I have described. They have discretionary authority, granted to them by licensing boards, to further the significant practical interest of the public in obtaining health care. They are therefore fiduciaries for the public in the very same way that a trustee of a charitable trust aimed at enhancing the public's literacy is a fiduciary. The pressure to narrow this conclusion to health care professionals who owe their income to the public is unwarranted.

Another objection is that the whole apparatus of fiduciary theory is unnecessary for understanding the duty I'm focused on, since one could explain it by appealing to some other factor instead: a simpler one, such as health care professionals' consent to do what their profession expects of them, or fair play. (On how consent and fair play can ground duties, see Chapter 5.) Could these professionals not have a duty to the public simply because they consented to it upon entering their profession, or because they receive (or have received) substantial benefits from the public, making it only fair that they demonstrate their loyalty to the public? In response, it is not at all clear that consent or fair play could provide the basis for this duty to the public. Consider, with respect to consent, that some health care professionals may not even know they have an obligation to the public or what

---

[33] I first heard this objection from Julian Savulescu in private conversation, who did not elaborate on it. The elaboration I give here comes from Andrew Botterell, who had the same objection.

this obligation entails, in which case they could not have properly consented to it. Or if they do know about this requirement, then they might assume—understandably given what professional associations tend to say about conscientious objection—that their conscience can override it when the two conflict. In that case, they would not have consented to the sort of duty to the public that I believe they have, which, as we'll see, is a duty that must take precedence over their conscience (which is not to say that it leaves no room for their conscience).

In my view, health care professionals' duty to the public rests on the type of relationship they have with the public: a fiduciary one. It is contingent neither on whether they have consented to promote public health and equitable access, nor on whether it is fair to expect that they will do so because of the many benefits they've received from the public. This second point is significant, because what is fair in this regard does not clearly support the duty. The reason is that the benefits these professionals obtain can vary significantly depending on how they are educated (i.e., in a private or a public institution), how long they have been in the profession (e.g., 10 months or 10 years), what their employment situation is (private practice or an employee of a public hospital), *etcetera* (Malm et al. 2008, 11–12). Even the benefit of having a monopoly, or near monopoly, over the provision of health care services is unequal for health care professionals who recently joined the profession compared to those who have been in it for years. The latter have reaped this benefit already, while the former have not. In short, what is fair given the benefits that health care professionals receive cannot explain a duty that is meant to apply to all of them equally.[34]

A final objection—the one that will encourage me to expand on my theory about these professionals being fiduciaries for the public—is that their duty of loyalty to the public is vague. I have suggested that it targets the collective health care interests of members of the public. But does it require that health care professionals provide treatment for every member of the public, or, more realistically, for every member who seeks treatment from them? If it did, then the view I'm developing now would conflict with what I said earlier, which is that individual health care professionals do not normally have a duty to treat everyone who seeks health care from them.

Thankfully, there is reason not to interpret the fiduciary duty of health care professionals to the public as a duty to treat everyone. Recall, the duty

---

[34] That is true, granted, unless there is a threshold of benefit that these professionals must reach before they could have the duty, and this threshold is set very low.

requires that they fulfill the public's *collective* interests (i.e., in equitable access to care and public health), not their individual interests. Notice also that for patients who do not yet have a health care professional of their own who could honor a request they have for service, being treated by a particular health care professional, as opposed to any health care professional, is usually an *individual* interest.[35] If I need orthopedic surgery, for example, having never had it before and hear that Dr. G is the best orthopedic surgeon in my city, then my interest in being treated by Dr. G is individual in nature. If the desire of prospective patients in being served by a particular health care professional is normally an individual interest, but the duty to the public targets only collective interests, then the duty cannot require that health care professionals welcome all prospective patients into their practice (i.e., welcome everyone who wants to be treated by *them* specifically). What then does the duty require of them? Surely, it cannot allow them to turn down prospective patients for just any reason, including because they feel like it. So how exactly are they meant to express their loyalty to the public?

I believe that we go a long way toward answering this question if we conceive of the duty as directed toward certain purposes (or ends)—specifically of enhancing public health and equitable access to care—rather than toward individual people, those to whom health care professionals might owe specific actions. This formulation allows us to limit the reasons they can have for turning down prospective patients to reasons that cohere with these purposes. A model of fiduciary loyalty as loyalty to purposes, not people, already exists in law and is generally used to understand the fiduciary duty of people who are fiduciaries for the public, such as trustees for charitable purpose trusts and CEOs of government corporations (Miller and Gold 2015).[36] These fiduciaries have what legal theorists call a "governance" mandate. I want to propose that the same sort of mandate exists for health care professionals in their relationship to the public.

---

[35] The exception is where the prospective patients have no alternative but to receive care from this particular health care professional. Perhaps the professional practices in a remote area, where very few health care professionals work. In that case, obtaining care from this person could be both a collective and an individual interest.

[36] The idea that duties could be directed toward certain purposes (or ends) is foreign neither to fiduciary law, nor to our moral thinking. With respect to the latter, consider that Kantian imperfect duties require that we adopt certain ends, rather than do specific things for specific people. Kant wrote of obligatory ends in the *Doctrine of Virtue*, including the end of others' happiness, which informs our imperfect duty to others (Kant 1797/1996, 4:430; see also Korsgaard 1996, Ch. 4).

A governance mandate occurs whenever fiduciaries are authorized to use their discretion to advance certain "abstract" purposes, such as literacy or public access to transportation. (To be clear, purposes count as abstract if they are not tied to—that is, they are abstracted away from—the interests of determinate individuals; Miller and Gold 2015, 517, 523.) By contrast, with a "service mandate," which is what health care professionals have (or can have) in their relationships with patients, the fiduciary is obligated to further the interests of specific individuals (2015, 521–2).[37] The purposes that define a governance mandate can involve aiding the public, but not serving individual members of it—not as individuals, not without the mandate being a service one.

The duties that attach to a governance mandate include a duty of loyalty, but again the loyalty is owed to purposes rather than to individual persons (Miller and Gold 2015). To be exact, fiduciaries with such a mandate owe their fidelity to the purpose(s) outlined in the mandate. They must exercise their "discretionary powers exclusively with a mind to advancing those purposes" (563), and thus must endeavor to avoid conflicts that might prevent them from exhibiting this loyalty while acting in their fiduciary capacity (see Chapter 5). Their mandate cannot tell them exactly how to express their loyalty, not without denying them the discretion that all fiduciaries possess, although it does demand that their actions be consistent with them being devoted to the relevant purposes. For example, a trustee who has a governance mandate to promote literacy must engage, as a trustee, only in actions that could serve this purpose, such as increasing awareness about the importance of literacy or providing resources to teachers for improving literacy.

Since the duty of loyalty that accompanies a governance mandate targets purposes, not persons, it does not correlate with a claim right of any person to the loyal pursuit of that person's individual interests. No such right exists, for instance, among individuals whose interests might be furthered by a government corporation that is responsible for public transportation. These individuals could legitimately criticize such an entity for failing to fulfill its public purpose, but not for neglecting their personal interests, such as an interest in having train service close to their home. To say that fiduciaries with a governance mandate are not accountable to individual persons (qua individuals) is not to say, however, that they are *unaccountable*. On the

---

[37] An example is the mandate of my family doctor to pursue my medical interests and those of my children. She, my doctor, has been empowered by me and my partner to act "in the service of" our family (Miller and Gold 2015, 521).

contrary, they can be expected to demonstrate their loyalty to "any of a number of persons or entities occupying a monitoring and enforcement role in respect of the mandate" (Miller and Gold 2015, 554). Examples include the benefactor of a charitable purpose trust, the government itself in the case of a government corporation, or a licensing board for health care professionals.

If indeed health care professionals' duty of loyalty to the public falls under a governance mandate, then we should understand the duty in the following way. It requires that these professionals be firmly committed to promoting public health and equitable access, and that this commitment be evident through their actions in their practice. If they rarely took on prospective patients, refused to accept those who are unlikely to receive the care they need otherwise, or just turned prospective patients away for no good reason, then they could not honestly say that they are committed to public health and equitable access. Moreover, they would not be fulfilling their duty to the public. At the same time, health care professionals do not have a duty to treat *all* members of the public or satisfy the interests of any individual member in being treated by them specifically. Being devoted to the purposes that define their mandate could actually require them to turn away prospective patients if taking them on would compromise their ability to care competently or safely for their existing patients, would involve them providing care that they deem to be futile, or the like (AMA 2016, 1.1.2).

To conclude, it is both useful and reasonable to think that the fiduciary duty health care professionals owe to the public to promote public health and equitable access to care is a duty to advance these purposes, which would make it part of a governance mandate. This theory is helpful not only in comprehending what it could mean for health care professionals to be loyal to the public, but also in understanding how their freedom of conscience should be limited outside of established relationships with patients. Let me turn to this final topic now.

2.1.2 Conscientious refusals

If health care professionals owe their fidelity to the purposes of public health and equitable access to care, then they cannot have unlimited freedom to choose on grounds of conscience which prospective patients to accept. This duty would require of those who wish to give prior notice of their conscientious objections, for example, that their notices direct prospective patients to alternative providers of the relevant services. At the same time, the duty could give health care professionals more leeway in expressing their conscience when it conflicts with what is standard of care than the duty of loyalty does that they have (or can have) toward their current patients. These are the claims I wish to argue for now.

First, let me explain why a fiduciary duty to the public should take precedence over a health care professional's conscience. My reasoning closely resembles that which I gave in Chapter 5 for why a fiduciary duty to one's own patients should trump one's conscience.[38] For consider that if it were the other way around—if conscience trumped the duty—then the duty would have to exist *prima facie* and only in the absence of conflict with one's conscience. Health care professionals cannot, however, be both fiduciaries and in possession of a right to conscience that allows them to ignore their fiduciary mandate—in this case, to promote public health and equitable access—whenever their conscience demands that they do so. For they could hardly be relied on to be loyal in that case, and yet the mandate clearly demands their loyalty.[39]

As I suggested above, health care professionals must have some leeway, however, in how they understand their mandate to serve the public. Could they not interpret it in a way that coheres with their conscience, even when their conscience tells them not to provide access to standard services (i.e., legal and professionally accepted services)? For example, pharmacists who morally object to the abortion pill might insist that by refusing to offer it or refer patients for it, they are promoting public health, understood by them to include the health of human embryos and fetuses. To respond to such an objection, particularly as it concerns typical refusals in reproductive health care, I seriously doubt that in jurisdictions where there is a legal right of access to abortion, the governance mandates of health care professionals grant them the authority to act in embryos' or fetuses' interests when those

[38] The reasoning applies, to be clear, regardless of whether the duty stems from a governance mandate or a service one.

[39] But one might ask, what if the mandate itself acknowledged that these professionals have a right to conscientious objection? In that case, it could not demand their loyalty to certain purposes *over* their conscience. For example, the Medical Board of Australia's *Good Medical Practice: A Code of Conduct for Doctors in Australia* states that they have a "right to not provide or directly participate in treatments to which [they] conscientiously object" (2014, 2.4.6). To respond to this objection, such a code would be internally inconsistent if it gave health care professionals a duty to promote public health and access to care—a duty that I have argued should be understood as fiduciary—along with an unlimited right to conscience. For the duty and the right, so understood, are simply incompatible with one another, as suggested in the previous paragraph. To be clear, this problem does not actually plague the code of the Medical Board of Australia, which qualifies the right I named above by stating that physicians must not use their conscientious objections "to impede access to treatments that are legal" (2.4.6) and must not allow their "moral or religious views to deny patients access to medical care" (2.4.7).

interests conflict with patients' reproductive freedom or health. For the mandates would then contradict the right to abortion access. What is more, the integrity of health care professions and public trust in them requires that health care professionals do not interpret their governance mandate through the lens of their (personal) conscience rather than in accordance with professional standards of care. I made similar claims in Chapter 5 with respect to the service mandates of health care professionals who act in a fiduciary capacity in their relationships with patients.

If these points are correct, then the discretion health care professionals have (or should have) in deciding how to promote public health and access to care does not extend to them violating the standards of care of their profession or defining the "public" so that it includes fetuses or embryos in unwanted pregnancies (i.e., in jurisdictions where services like abortions are, in fact, legal). Such conduct conflicts with these professionals being loyal to the purposes of enhancing public health and equitable access. When conflicts like these occur, moreover, health care professionals' loyalty should win out over their conscience, or so I have argued. Now what does this mean in concrete terms? What does it entail specifically for health care professionals who wish to give prior notice of their conscientious refusals? Let me home in on these cases and then make a more general statement about how loyalty to the public restricts any right health care professionals have to make conscientious objections outside of established relationships with patients.

Assuming that giving prior notice of a conscientious objection is even ethical,[40] fidelity to the purpose of equitable access requires that objectors direct prospective patients to alternative sources of access to the care these people need, or at least to alternative sources of information about access. It is not enough to write that the health care professional on call will not prescribe the birth control pill or perform any other standard service. Rather, in addition, the notice should refer people to health care professionals nearby who are willing and able to offer the relevant service or include contact details for an organization (e.g., Planned Parenthood) that itself will give referrals of this kind. Objectors who ignore such a requirement when publicizing their objections are not being loyal to the purposes that define their mandate towards the public. They are prioritizing their conscience over their duty of loyalty to the public, which, as I've explained, is morally inappropriate. In general, health care professionals demonstrate this loyalty by ensuring that

---

[40] I question this assumption earlier, in Section 1.2.

the people who approach them wanting health care understand where else they can obtain it nearby if they, the professionals, cannot or will not provide it. Furthermore, if there are no alternative sources of access in their area, then the professionals themselves should complain to their profession, whom I have said must share with them the burden of promoting equitable access. At the same time, when health care professionals' only reason for refusing access to prospective patients is conscience, and no other health care professionals are available to do what they morally object to do, then they should, out of fidelity to their mandate, do it anyway.[41] In demanding such action, along with referrals for treatments that objectors deem to be morally offensive, the mandate restricts their freedom of conscience significantly.

So health care professionals' duty of loyalty to the public limits their conscience-based freedom to turn prospective patients away; but does it eliminate this freedom entirely? I think the answer is no. The reason is that there can be multiple avenues available for these professionals to fulfill the purposes of furthering public health and access to care, and when some avenues cohere with their conscience (to some degree at least), they can retain some freedom to act on it. Let me illustrate with gynecologists whose views about the sanctity of human life make them morally opposed to standard abortion services. They could show their fidelity to the purpose of supporting access to these services (which should be among the standard services they provide as gynecologists) by acceding to requests by prospective patients for them, by giving these patients proper referrals for them, or by working in a setting where new patients could obtain these services while having little to no contact with them, the objecting gynecologists. These professionals would, in all likelihood, violate their conscience if they chose the first two options, but not if they chose the last. To elaborate on it, the setting could be a large hospital where others will normally be available to do the intake of patients wanting an abortion, and the hospital respects the moral decisions of anti-abortion health care professionals not to be involved with these patients. If our gynecologists chose to work in this way in this environment, then I don't think they would be shirking their duty to further equitable access to care. On the contrary, a decision like this would conform to the duty since the hospital itself provides access to abortions; they could

---

[41] This point appears in the model policy for conscientious objections in medicine that I developed with Jocelyn Downie and Jacquelyn Shaw (2013, 31; section 5.4).

have chosen instead to work at an institution that severely inhibits this access and would insist they do the same.

If this last part is correct, then there can be—and one might argue, *should* be—options available to conscientious objectors that could allow them to abide by their conscience while fulfilling their fiduciary duty to the public. That is true even of health care professionals who conscientiously object to providing referrals for services that morally offend them. By contrast, the fiduciary duty of loyalty that health care professionals have (or may have) to their individual patients requires them to offer these patients, at the very least, referrals for services that the professionals conscientiously object to, regardless of whether they also object to the referrals (see Chapter 5). The upshot is that these professionals can have more freedom of conscience outside of fiduciary relationships with patients than inside of them.

I have endeavored to explain how health care professionals' duty to the public could be compatible with them exercising some freedom to turn down prospective patients for reasons of conscience, although I have focused mainly on how and why the duty restricts this conscience-based freedom. As a fiduciary duty that demands their fidelity to the purposes of public health and equitable access, it does not allow them to have unlimited freedom of this sort.

3. Conclusion

My main goal in this chapter has been to show that health care professionals' freedom to choose prospective patients on grounds of conscience must be significantly restricted. However, a further objective has been to describe and clarify my position on different "conscience-based" freedoms in health care. These include the freedoms to choose how to serve and whom to serve, where the latter entails the freedom to begin or end relationships with patients. In my view, these relationships are morally salient when they are fiduciary in nature, since what conscientious objectors are morally required to do can vary depending on whether they are objecting inside or outside of a fiduciary relationship with a patient. In addition, what explains what they are morally required to do will differ depending on this feature of the context they are in. Inside a fiduciary relationship with a specific patient, they have a duty to engage in the loyal pursuit of the patient's individual interests, while outside of such a relationship, they have a duty of loyalty to the public to further certain "purposes": public health and equitable access to care. Although the first duty may limit their freedom of conscience more than the second, the second duty is still demanding. It precludes health care professionals from allowing their conscience to dictate who becomes their patient in circumstances where they cannot ensure (e.g., by giving proper referrals) that prospective patients will receive the health care they need.

Conclusion

The interests of patients in receiving standard services should therefore be prioritized over the conscience of health care professionals. This book has defended this prioritizing approach over the compromise approach, which is dominant in bioethics. It has also focused on what I've called "typical refusals" in reproductive health care—especially, refusals to offer abortions or so-called "abortifacients"—because of a global trend of health care professionals engaging in such conduct (IWHC 2017; Chavkin et al. 2013). In countries where individuals or members of groups like the International Women's Health Coalition have fought hard to liberalize abortion laws, conscientious objection is limiting access to legal and safe abortions. My objective has been to philosophically support the view of the IWHC and others that laws or policies permitting this sort of behavior by health care professionals are morally unjustified.

The moral framework I've developed to defend the prioritizing approach to conscientious refusals is a fiduciary one. I have maintained that normatively speaking, health care professionals—those who are charged with gatekeeping access to health care services—are fiduciaries both for their patients and for the public they are licensed to serve. In this capacity, they have discretionary authority to act on behalf of these beneficiaries and must use this power to promote their beneficiaries' interests rather than other interests including the professionals' own. Relevant interests of their patients are in health (or health care), and of the public, in public health and equitable access to care. These concerns of patients and the public must take priority over the desire conscientious objectors have to act on their conscience, because that is what the fiduciary duty of loyalty requires. The fiduciary lens being applied here is relatively new to the bioethics literature, which includes statements to the effect that health care professionals (especially physicians) are fiduciaries for their patients, but which says relatively little about what that entails and nothing about how health care professionals could be fiduciaries for the public as a whole. My goal has been to show that applying the fiduciary framework to the issue of conscientious refusals is both appropriate

Conscience in Reproductive Health Care: Prioritizing Patient Interests. Carolyn McLeod, Oxford University Press (2020).
© Carolyn McLeod.
DOI: 10.1093/oso/9780198732723.001.0001

and illuminating. It can be illuminating as well, I assume, for other topics in bioethics, including conscientious conduct by health care professionals that does not amount to a conscientious refusal (e.g., conscientious commitment; see the Introduction).[1]

Like the report of the IWHC (2017), this book has concentrated on conscientious *refusal* (or objection) as a barrier to patients' receiving basic reproductive health services. I have interpreted this conduct primarily as a refusal to honor a request by a patient for a service that is both legal and professionally accepted. Abortion is an example in countries where abortion is legal and the standard of care for patients in an unwanted pregnancy is to be offered an abortion. I have argued in favor of taking the prioritizing approach to regulating both typical and atypical conscientious refusals, even when the latter are motivated by anti-oppressive values and even though this strategy is not perfect for these cases.

My analysis as a whole pertains to the conduct of health care professionals who are acting in their capacity as health care professionals and within fiduciary relationships with patients and the public. Outside of these contexts, health care professionals should have freedom of conscience that is as extensive as the freedom enjoyed by other citizens.[2] I have suggested that they should be free to voice their conscience with impunity in professional meetings, for example, or in other venues where professional policies get made. No matter the restrictions on their freedom of conscience within fiduciary relationships, health care professionals should always have opportunities for conscientious conduct that resists professional norms, which we know can be corrupt (as they were, e.g., in Nazi Germany). Thus, my view is not that these professionals should just accept whatever norms or policies are in place for their profession and never work to try to change them. My concern is, again, with conscientious *refusals*, which themselves don't even aim at policy change,[3] and which I've argued are morally impermissible, particularly

---

[1] See Chapter 5 on how this framework can be helpful in analyzing any conscientious conduct that patients themselves authorize. See Ryman (2017) on how illuminating it can be with respect to the ethics of commercial surrogacy, especially physicians' involvement in surrogacy arrangements.

[2] I have said that at times, however, while exercising this freedom, they may have to act in their capacity as a citizen rather than as a health care professional.

[3] Rather, their purpose is to seek protection for conscience (see the Introduction).

within established (fiduciary) relationships with patients.[4] This sort of conduct by health care professionals should not be protected.

In the end, I hope not only to have successfully defended the prioritizing approach, but also to have revealed the complexity of the moral issue of whether to protect conscience in health care, especially reproductive health care. Like those who support the compromise approach, I have recognized that conscientious tend to generate moral conflicts (resolvable ones). That is true because important interests are at stake for the objectors themselves and for the patients seeking care. I have added to our understanding about what the relevant interests are for patients who are denied abortions or contraception, and also for conscientious objectors. I have argued that the ability of health care professionals to act on their conscience can have moral value and *does* have this value when their conscience is dynamic rather than fixed, meaning that it responds to new moral knowledge they have gained.

Because of their moral complexity, I doubt that any solution to the problem of how to regulate conscientious refusals will be perfect. As I've said, the prioritizing approach is not perfect for dealing with atypical refusals that are motivated by anti-oppressive values (see Chapter 5, Section 3.3).[5] Perhaps we could try to prevent conscientious refusals from occurring altogether by imparting moral knowledge to health care professionals—for example, about the harm of denying patients access to abortions—with the hope that their conscience will align with what are (good) standards of care. Yet even with this knowledge, some health care professionals will continue to conscientiously object. They will also have to violate their conscience repeatedly in order to "stay in the game" (Prieur 2004), if the policies I have recommended are put in place (see Chapter 6). This fact, which is not morally insignificant,[6] should generate some moral discomfort in us (if only a small amount). I do not pretend that by taking the prioritizing approach, we should all feel completely morally settled, however. No strategy for regulating conscientious refusals will do that for us, again because of their moral complexity.

[4] I have made allowances for some conscientious objecting behavior that health care professionals engage in with prospective patients. See Chapter 6, Section 2.1.2.
[5] I have in mind here, in particular, the cases in Chapter 5 where I had to "bite the bullet" and say that the relevant refusal is morally problematic.
[6] That is true because there is personal value in leading a morally authentic life. See Chapter 1.

It is clear nevertheless that conscientious objectors should be governed by policies that conform to the prioritizing approach, rather than the compromise one. Health activists, such as members of the IWHC, should continue to fight for these policies because they take seriously the misuse or abuse of power that occurs with most conscientious refusals. The alternative of having permissive regulations on these refusals, especially those that target abortion and contraception, is something we should all resist.

Bibliography

Alford, C. F. 2001. *Whistleblowers: Broken Lives and Organizational Power*. Ithaca: Cornell University Press.

Almassi, B. 2014. Trust and the Duty of Organ Donation, *Bioethics* 28(6): 275–83.

Alvarez, M. 2016. Reasons for Action: Justification, Motivation, Explanation. In the *Stanford Encyclopedia of Philosophy*. Ed. E. Zalta. Retrieved on Nov. 23, 2017 at https://plato.stanford.edu/entries/reasons-just-vs-expl/.

American Medical Association (AMA). 2016. Code of Medical Ethics. Retrieved on June13,2019athttps://www.ama-assn.org/delivering-care/ethics/code-medical-ethics-overview.

Anonymous/xojane. 2015. I Was Pro-Life until I Accidentally Got Pregnant and Wanted an Abortion, *Alternet*. March 25. Retrieved on June 13, 2019 at https://www.alternet.org/belief/i-was-pro-life-until-i-accidentally-got-pregnant-and-wanted-abortion.

Appiah, A. 1990. Racisms. In *Anatomy of Racism*. Ed. D. T. Goldberg. Minneapolis: University of Minnesota Press. Pp. 3–17.

Arras, J. D. 1988. The Fragile Web of Responsibility: AIDS and the Duty to Treat, *Hastings Center Report* 18(2): S10–20.

Austin, Z., P. A. Gregory, and J. C. Martin. 2006. Characterizing the Professional Relationships of Community Pharmacists, *Research in Social and Administrative Pharmacy* 2(4): 533–46.

Australian Medical Association. 2016. Code of Ethics 2004 (Revised 2016). Retrieved on June 13, 2019 at https://ama.com.au/media/new-code-ethics-doctors.

Baergen, R. and C. Owens. 2006. Revisiting Pharmacists' Refusals to Dispense Emergency Contraception, *Obstetrics & Gynecology* 108(5): 1277–82.

Baier, A. 1986. Trust and Anti-trust, *Ethics* 96: 231–60.

Bartky, S. L. 1990. On Psychological Oppression. In her *Femininity and Domination: Studies in the Phenomenology of Oppression*. New York, NY: Routledge. Pp. 22–32.

Bayles, M. D. 1988. The Professional–Client Relationship. In *Ethical Issues in Professional Life*. Ed. J. C. Callahan. Oxford: Oxford University Press. Pp. 113–20.

Baylis, F. 1993. Assisted Reproductive Technologies: Informed Choice. In New Reproductive Technologies: Ethical Aspects. *Vol. 1 of the Research Studies of the Royal Commission on New Reproductive Technologies*. Ottawa: Minister of Supply and Services Canada.

Benjamin, M. 1990. *Splitting the Difference: Compromise and Integrity in Ethics and Politics*. Lawrence, KA: University of Kansas Press.

Benjamin, M. 1995. Conscience. In the *Encyclopedia of Bioethics*, Vol. 1. Ed. W. T. Reich. 2nd ed. Basingstoke: Macmillan. Pp. 469–72.

Benjamin, M. and J. Curtis. 1992. *Ethics in Nursing*. 3rd ed. New York: Oxford University Press.

Ben-Moshe, N. 2019. The Truth Behind Conscientious Objection in Medicine, *Journal of Medical Ethics* 45(6): 404–410.

Benson, P. 2000. Feeling Crazy: Self-worth and the Social Character of Responsibility. In *Relational Autonomy: Feminist Perspectives on Autonomy, Agency, and the Social Self*. Ed. C. Mackenzie and N. Stoljar. Oxford: Oxford University Press. Pp. 72–93.

Blake, V. 2012. When Is a Patient-Physician Relationship Established? *The Virtual Mentor* 14(5): 403–6.

Blustein, J. 1993. Doing What the Patient Orders: Maintaining Integrity in the Doctor–Patient Relationship, *Bioethics* 7: 289–314.

Botterell, A. and C. McLeod. 2015. Can a Right to Reproduce Justify the Status Quo on Parental Licensing? In *Permissible Progeny: The Morality of Procreation and Parenting*. Ed. R. Vernon, S. Hannan, and S. Brennan. New York: Oxford University Press. Pp. 184–207.

Brock, D. 2008. Conscientious Refusals by Physicians and Pharmacists: Who Is Obligated to Do What, and Why? *Theoretical Medicine & Bioethics* 29: 187–200.

Brownlee, K. 2012. *Conscience and Conviction: The Case for Civil Disobedience*. Oxford: Oxford University Press.

Brownlee, K. 2013. Civil Disobedience. In the *Stanford Encyclopedia of Philosophy*. Ed. E. Zalta. Originally published 2007. Retrieved on June 13, 2019 at https://plato.stanford.edu/entries/civil-disobedience/.

Buchbinder, M., D. Lassiter, R. Mercier, A. Bryant, and A. D. Lyerly. 2016. Reframing Conscientious Care: Providing Abortion Care When Law and Conscience Collide, *Hastings Center Report* 46(2): 22–30.

Calhoun, C. 1995. Standing for Something, *The Journal of Philosophy* 92: 235–60.

Canadian Association of Midwives. 2015. The Canadian Midwifery Model of Care Position Statement. Retrieved on June 13, 2019 at https://canadianmidwives.org/wp-content/uploads/2016/06/CAM-MoCPSFINAL-OCT2015-ENG-FINAL.pdf.

Canadian Medical Association. 2017. CMA Policy: Medical Assistance in Dying. Retrieved on June 13, 2019 at https://policybase.cma.ca/documents/Policypdf/PD17-03.pdf.

Canadian Medical Association. 2018. CMA Code of Ethics and Professionalism. Retrieved on June 13, 2019 at https://policybase.cma.ca/documents/policypdf/PD19-03.pdf.

Canadian Nurses Association. 2017. Code of Ethics for Registered Nurses. Retrieved on June 13, 2019 at https://www.cna-aiic.ca/~/media/cna/page-content/pdf-en/code-of-ethics-2017-edition-secure-interactive.

Cannold, L. 1994. Consequence for Patients of Health Care Professionals' Conscientious Actions: The Ban on Abortions in South Australia, *Journal of Medical Ethics* 20: 80–6.

Cantor, J. and K. Baum. 2004. The Limits of Conscientious Objection—May Pharmacists Refuse to Fill Prescriptions for Emergency Contraception? *New England Journal of Medicine* 351(19): 2008–12.

Card, C. 1996. Responsibility and Moral Luck. In her *The Unnatural Lottery: Character and Moral Luck*. Philadelphia: Temple University Press. Pp. 21–48.

Card, R. F. 2007. Conscientious Objection and Emergency Contraception, *American Journal of Bioethics* 7(6): 8–14.

Caro, N. dir. 2005. North Country. [film] Participant Productions et al.

Chavkin, W., L. Leitman, and K. Polin. 2013. Conscientious Objection and Refusal to Provide Reproductive Healthcare: A White Paper Examining Prevalence, Health Consequences, and Policy Responses, *International Journal of Gynecology and Obstetrics* 123: S41–56.

Chavkin, W., L. Swerdlow, and J. Fifield. 2017. Regulation of Conscientious Objection to Abortion: An International Comparative Multiple-case Study, *Health and Human Rights* 19(1): 55–68.

Chervenak, F. A. and L. B. McCullough. 2008. The Ethics of Direct and Indirect Referral for Termination of Pregnancy, *American Journal of Obstetrics and Gynecology* 199(3): 232.e1–3.

Childress, J. 1979. Appeals to Conscience, *Ethics* 89(4): 315–35.

Childress, J. 1997. Conscience and Conscientious Actions in the Context of MCOs, *Kennedy Institute of Ethics Journal* 7: 403–11.

Childress, J. 2006. Exploring Claims to Conscience. A Presentation at the Conference, "Should Conscience Be Your Guide? Exploring Conscience-based Refusals in Health Care." Held June 20, at the University of Maryland School of Law.

Chin, J. J. 2002. Doctor–Patient Relationship: From Medical Paternalism to Enhanced Autonomy, *Singapore Medical Journal* 43(3): 152–5.

Clark, C. C. 2002. Trust in Medicine, *Journal of Medicine and Philosophy* 27(1): 11–29.

Clark, C. C. 2005. In Harm's Way: AMA Physicians and the Duty to Treat, *Journal of Medicine and Philosophy* 30: 65–87.

Coady, C. A. J. 2016. Kimberley Brownlee: *Conscience and Conviction: The Case for Civil Disobedience*, *Journal of Value Inquiry* 50: 501–6.

Cockrill, K. and A. Nack. 2013. "I'm Not That Type of Person": Managing the Stigma of Having an Abortion, *Deviant Behavior* 34(12): 973–90.

Cockrill, K., U. D. Upadhyay, and D. G. Foster. 2013. The Stigma of Having an Abortion: Development of a Scale and Characteristics of Women Experiencing Abortion Stigma, *Perspectives on Sexual and Reproductive Health* 45(2): 79–88.

Cogley, Z. 2012. Trust and the Trickster Problem, *Analytic Philosophy* 53(1): 30–47.

Conaglen, M. 2010. *Fiduciary Loyalty: Protecting the Due Performance of Non-fiduciary Duties*. Oxford: Hart Publishing.

Conly, S. 2013. *Against Autonomy: Justifying Coercive Paternalism*. New York: Cambridge University Press.

Cowley, C. 2015. A Defense of Conscientious Objection in Medicine: A Reply to Schuklenk and Savulescu, *Bioethics* 30(5): 358–64.

Criddle, E. J. and E. Fox Decent. 2018. Guardians of Legal Order: The Dual Commissions of Public Authorities. In *Fiduciary Government*. Ed. E. J. Criddle,

E. Fox-Decent, P. B. Miller, A. Gold, S. H. Kim. Cambridge: Cambridge University Press. Pp. 67–95.

Croxatto, H. B., V. Brache, M. Pavez, et al. 2004. Pituitary–ovarian Function Following the Standard Levonorgestrel Emergency Contraceptive Dose or a Single 0.75-mg. Dose Given on the Days Preceding Ovulation, *Contraception* 70: 442–50.

Davidoff, F. 2006. Sex, Politics, and Morality at the FDA: Reflections on the Plan B Decision, *Hastings Center Report* 36(2): 20–5.

Davion, V. 1991. Integrity and Radical Change. In *Feminist Ethics*. Ed. C. Card. Lawrence, KA: University of Kansas Press. Pp. 180–92.

Davison, G., J. Hirst, and S. Macintyre. 2003. Canberra. In *The Oxford Companion to Australian History (online)*. Oxford: Oxford University Press.

DesAutels, P. 2009. Resisting Organizational Power. In *Feminist Ethics and Social and Political Philosophy: Theorizing the Non-ideal*. Ed. L. Tessman. Dordrecht: Springer. Pp. 223–36.

Dickens, B. M. 2008. Conscientious Commitment, *The Lancet* 371(9620): P1240–1.

Dickens, B. M. and R. J. Cook. 2011. Conscientious Commitment to Women's Health, *International Journal of Gynaecology and Obstetrics* 113(2): 163–6.

Downie, J. 2012. Resistance Is Essential: Relational Responses to Recent Law and Policy Initiatives Involving Reproduction. In *Being Relational: Reflections on Relational Theory and Health Law and Policy*. Ed. J. Downie and J. Lewellyn. Vancouver: University of British Columbia Press. Pp. 209–29.

Downie, J., C. McLeod, and J. Shaw. 2013. Moving forward with a Clear Conscience: A Model of Conscientious Objection Policy for Canadian Colleges of Physicians and Surgeons, *Health Law Review* 21(3): 28–32.

Downie, J. and C. Nassar. 2008. Barriers to Access to Abortion through a Legal Lens, *Health Law Journal* 15: 143–73.

Dunn, S. and M. Brooks. 2018. Mifepristone, *CMAJ* June 4, 190(22): E688.

Easterbrook, F. H. and D. R. Fischel. 1991. *The Economic Structure of Corporate Law*. Cambridge, MA: Harvard University Press.

Emanuel, E. J. and L. L. Emanuel. 1992. Four Models of the Physician–Patient Relationship, *Journal of the American Medical Association* 267(16): 22–9.

Erdely, S. R. 2007. Doctors' Beliefs Hinder Patient Care, *Self Magazine*, June. Retrieved on June 13, 2019 at http://www.nbcnews.com/id/19190916/ns/health-womens_health/#.VWNSv2Ak9oM.

Fairhurst, K, S. Ziebland, S. Wyke, P. Seaman, and A. Glasier. 2004. Emergency Contraception: Why Can't You Give It Away? Qualitative Findings from an Evaluation of Advance Provision of Emergency Contraception, *Contraception* 70: 25–9.

Fausto-Sterling, A. 2000. *Sexing the Body: Gender Politics and the Construction of Sexuality*. New York: Basic Books.

Feinberg, J. 1984. *The Moral Limits of the Criminal Law, Volume One: Harm to Others*. New York: Oxford University Press.

Fenton, E. and L. Lomasky. 2005. Dispensing with Liberty: Conscientious Refusal and the "Morning-after Pill," *Journal of Medicine and Philosophy* 30: 579–92.

Fiala, C. and J. H. Arthur. 2017. There Is No Defence for "Conscientious Objection" in Reproductive Health Care, *European Journal of Obstetrics & Gynecology and Reproductive Biology* 216: 254–8.

Fiala, C., K. G. Danielsson, O. Heikinheimo, J. A. Guðmundsson and J. Arthur. 2016. Yes We Can! Successful Examples of Disallowing "Conscientious Objection" in Reproductive Health Care, *The European Journal of Contraception & Reproductive Health Care* 21(3): 201–6.

Finer, L. B., L. F. Frohwirth, L. A. Dauphinee, S. Singh, and A. M. Moore. 2005. Reasons U.S. Women Have Abortions: Quantitative and Qualitative Perspectives, *Perspectives on Sexual and Reproductive Health* 37(3): 110–18.

Fox Decent, E. 2005. The Fiduciary Nature of State Legal Authority, *Queen's Law Journal* 31: 259–310.

Free, C., R. M. Lee, and J. Ogden. 2002. Young Women's Accounts of Factors Influencing their Use and Non-use of Emergency Contraception: In-depth Interview Study, *British Medical Journal* 325(7377): 1393–6.

Frye, M. 1983. Oppression. In her *The Politics of Reality: Essays in Feminist Theory.* Freedom, CA: Crossing Press. Pp. 1–16.

FSRH (Faculty of Sexual and Reproductive Healthcare of the Royal College of Obstetricians and Gynaecologists, UK). 2017. Emergency Contraception. Retrieved June 14, 2019 at https://www.fsrh.org/news/fsrh-launches-new-emergency-contraception-guideline/.

Gee, R. E. 2006. Plan B, Reproductive Rights, and Physician Activism, *New England Journal of Medicine* 355(1): 4, 5.

Gemzell-Danielsson, K., C. Berger, and P. G. Lalitkumar. 2014. Mechanisms of Action of Oral Emergency Contraception, *Gynecological Endocrinology* 30(10): 685–7.

Gilbert, D. 2006. *Stumbling on Happiness.* New York: Knopf.

Gold, A. and P. Miller, eds. 2014. *Philosophical Foundations of Fiduciary Law.* Oxford: Oxford University Press.

Gold, R. B. and E. Nash. 2007. State Abortion Counseling Policies and the Fundamental Principles of Informed Consent, *Guttmacher Policy Review* 10(4): 6–13.

Greenberger, M. D. and R. Vogelstein. 2005. Pharmacist Refusals: A Threat to Women's Health, *Science* 308(5728): 1557–8.

Grimes, D. A., J. Benson, S. Singh, M. Romero, B. Ganatra, F. E. Okonofua, and I. H. Shah. 2006. Unsafe Abortion: The Preventable Pandemic, *The Lancet* 368(9550): 1908–19.

Guibilini, A. 2014. The Paradox of Conscientious Objection and the Anemic Concept of "Conscience": Downplaying the Role of Moral Integrity in Health Care, *Kennedy Institute of Ethics Journal* 24(2): 159–85.

Haddad, L. B. and N. M. Nour. 2009. Unsafe Abortion: Unnecessary Maternal Mortality, *Reviews in Obstetrics & Gynecology* 2(2): 122–6.

Harding, M. 2016. Fiduciary Undertakings. In *Contract, Status, and Fiduciary Law.* Ed. P. B. Miller and A. S. Gold. Oxford: Oxford University Press. Pp. 71–90.

Harries, J., D. Cooper, A. Strebel, and C. J. Colvin. 2014. Conscientious Objection and its Impact on Abortion Service Provision in South Africa: A Qualitative Study, *Reproductive Health* 11(1): 11–16.

Harwood, K. 2009. Egg Freezing: A Breakthrough for Reproductive Autonomy? *Bioethics* 32(1): 39–46.

Hill Jr., T. E. 1998. Four Conceptions of Conscience. In *Integrity and Conscience*. Ed. I. Shapiro and R. Adams. New York: New York University Press. Pp. 13–52.

Holcombe, S. J., A. Berhe, and A. Cherie. 2015. Personal Beliefs and Professional Responsibilities: Ethiopian Midwives' Attitudes toward Providing Abortion Services after Legal Reform, *Studies in Family Planning* 46(1): 73–95.

Holton, R. 1994. Deciding to Trust, Coming to Believe, *Australasian Journal of Philosophy* 72(1): 63–76.

Horsburgh, H. J. N. 1960. The Ethics of Trust, *Philosophical Quarterly* 10: 343–54.

Howard, D. S. 2013. On Behalf of Another. PhD Dissertation (Philosophy). Brown University.

Hursthouse, R. 1999. *On Virtue Ethics*. Oxford: Oxford University Press.

International Pharmaceutical Federation/Federation Internationale Pharmaceutique. 2014. FIP Statement of Professional Standards: Codes of Ethics for Pharmacists. Retrieved on June 15, 2019 at http://apps.who.int/medicinedocs/documents/s19757en/s19757en.pdf.

International Women's Health Coalition (IWHC). 2017. Unconscionable: When Providers Deny Abortion Care. Retrieved June 14, 2019 at https://iwhc.org/resources/unconscionable-when-providers-deny-abortion-care/.

Jacoby, B. 2011. Trust and Betrayal: A Conceptual Analysis. PhD Dissertation (Philosophy), Macquarie University.

Joffe, C. 2013. The Politicization of Abortion and the Evolution of Abortion Counseling, *American Journal of Public Health* 103(1): 57–65.

Jones, K. 1996. Trust as an Affective Attitude, *Ethics* 107(1): 4–25.

Jones, K. 2012. Trustworthiness, *Ethics* 123(1): 61–85.

Jones, P. 2016. Group Rights. In the *Stanford Encyclopedia of Philosophy*. Ed. E. Zalta. Retrieved on June 13, 2019 at https://plato.stanford.edu/entries/rights-group/.

Kamm, F. M. 2007. *Intricate Ethics: Rights, Responsibilities, and Permissible Harm*. Oxford: Oxford University Press.

Kant, I. 1784/1996. What Is Enlightenment? In *Practical Philosophy*. Trans. and ed. M. J. Gregor. Cambridge: Cambridge University Press.

Kant, I. 1797/1996. Doctrine of the Elements of Ethics, Part I (The Doctrine of Virtue). In *The Metaphysics of Morals*. Trans. and ed. M. J. Gregor. Cambridge: Cambridge University Press.

Kantymir, L. and C. McLeod. 2014. Justification for Conscience Exemptions in Health Care, In C. McLeod and J. Downie, eds. *Let Conscience Be their Guide? Conscientious Refusals in Health Care*. Special issue of *Bioethics* 28(1): 16–23.

Kapp, N., D. Grossman, E. Jackson, L. Castleman, and D. Brahmi. 2017. A Research Agenda for Moving Early Medical Pregnancy Termination over the Counter, *BJOG: An International Journal of Obstetrics & Gynaecology* 124(11): https://doi.org/10.1111/1471-0528.14646.

Kimport, K., K. Foster, and T. A. Weitz. 2011. Social Sources of Women's Emotional Difficulty after Abortion: Lessons from Women's Abortion Narratives, *Perspectives on Sexual and Reproductive Health* 43(2): 103–9.

Kiss, E. 1998. Conscience and Moral Psychology: Reflections on Thomas Hill's "Four Conceptions of Conscience." In *Integrity and Conscience*. Ed. I. Shapiro and R. Adams. New York: New York University Press. Pp. 69–76.

Kittay, E. F. 1999. *Love's Labor: Essays on Women, Equality, and Dependency*. New York: Routledge.

Kelleher, P. 2010. Emergency Contraception and Conscientious Objection, *Journal of Applied Philosophy* 27(3): 290–304.

Kennett, J. 2017. The Cost of Conscience: Kant on Conscience and Conscientious Objection, *Cambridge Quarterly of Healthcare Ethics* 26: 69–81.

Koegh, L. A., L. Gilliam, M. Bismark, K. McNamee, A. Webster, C. Bayly, and D. Newton. 2019. Conscientious Objection to Abortion, the Law and its Implementation in Victoria, Australia: Perspectives of Abortion Service Providers, *BMC Medical Ethics* 20(11): https://doi.org/10.1186/S12910-019-0346-1.

Kolers, A. 2014. Am I My Profession's Keeper? In C. McLeod and J. Downie, eds. *Let Conscience Be their Guide? Conscientious Refusals in Health Care*. Special issue of *Bioethics* 28(1): 1–7.

Korsgaard, C. M. 1996. *Creating the Kingdom of Ends*. Cambridge: Cambridge University Press.

Krishnan, M. 2014. Calgary Doctor Refuses to Prescribe Birth Control over Moral Beliefs, *Calgary Herald*. June 27. Retrieved on June 13, 2019 at http://www.calgaryherald.com/news/calgary/Calgary+doctor+refuses+prescribe+birth+control+over+moral+beliefs/9978442/story.html.

Kultgen, J. 2014. Professional Paternalism, *Ethical Theory and Moral Practice* 17: 399–412.

Kumar, A., L. Hessini, and E. M. Mitchell. 2009. Conceptualising Abortion Stigma, *Culture, Health & Sexuality* 11(6): 625–39.

Laby, A. B. 2008. The Fiduciary Obligation as the Adoption of Ends, *Buffalo Law Review* 56(1): 99–167.

Lahno, B. 2001. On the Emotional Character of Trust, *Ethical Theory and Moral Practice* 4(2): 171–89.

Langbein, J. H. 1995. The Contractarian Basis of the Law of Trusts, *Yale Law Journal* 105: 625–75.

Laugminas, S. G. 2005. Pharmacists Battling Lawsuits over Conscience Issues, *National Catholic Register* Feb. 13–19. Retrieved on June 13, 2019 at: https://www.consciencelaws.org/background/procedures/birth009.aspx.

Laurance, J. 2007. Abortion Crisis as Doctors Refuse to Perform Surgery, *The Independent* April 16.

Lepora, C. 2012. On Compromise and Being Compromised, *Journal of Political Philosophy* 20 (1): 1–22.

Levins Morales, A. 1998. *Medicine Stories: History, Culture and the Politics of Integrity*. Cambridge, MA: South End Press.

Liberman, A. 2017. Wrongness, Responsibility, and Conscientious Refusals in Health Care, *Bioethics* 31(7): 495–504.

Little, M. O. 1999. Abortion, Intimacy, and the Duty to Gestate, *Ethical Theory and Moral Practice* 2: 295–312.

Lucero II, L. 2018. Walgreens Pharmacist Denies Woman with Unviable Pregnancy the Medication Needed to End It, *New York Times*, June 25. Retrieved on June 14, 2019athttps://www.nytimes.com/2018/06/25/us/walgreens-pharmacist-pregnancy-miscarriage.html.

Lyerly, A. D. and M. O. Little. 2013. The Limits of Conscientious Refusal: A Duty to Ensure Access, *The Virtual Mentor: American Medical Association Journal of Ethics* 15(3): 257–62.

Lyerly, A. D., M. O. Little, and R. R. Faden. 2008. A Critique of the Fetus as Patient, *The American Journal of Bioethics* 8(7): 42–6.

Lynch, H. F. 2008. *Conflicts of Conscience in Health Care: An Institutional Compromise*. Cambridge, MA: MIT Press.

Macfarlane, U. dir. 2008. *Abortion: The Choice. [documentary]* Century Films et al.

Mackenzie, C. and N. Stoljar. 2000. Introduction: Autonomy Refigured. In their *Relational Autonomy: Feminist Perspectives on Autonomy, Agency, and the Social Self*. New York: Oxford. Pp. 3–31.

MacKinnon, B.-J. 2017. Abortion Pill Now Available for Free to Women in New Brunswick, *CBC News*, July 7. Retrieved on June 14, 2019 at https://www.cbc.ca/news/canada/new-brunswick/abortion-pill-mifegymiso-new-brunswick-free-1.4194436.

Malm, H., T. May, L. P. Francis, S. B. Omer, D. A. Salmon, and R. Hood. 2008. Ethics, Pandemics, and the Duty to Treat, *The American Journal of Bioethics* 8(8): 4–19.

Margalit, A. 2010. *On Compromise and Rotten Compromises*. Princeton: Princeton University Press.

Markovits, D. 2014. Sharing Ex Ante and Sharing Ex Post: The Non-Contractual Basis of Fiduciary Relations. In *Philosophical Foundations of Fiduciary Law*. Ed. P. B. Miller and A. S. Gold. Oxford: Oxford University Press. Pp. 209–24.

Marsh, J. 2014. Conscientious Refusals and Reason-Giving, *Bioethics* 28(6): 313–19.

Marshall, T. and A. McLaren. 2013. Henry Morgentaler. *The Canadian Encyclopedia*. Retrieved on June 13, 2019 at http://www.thecanadianencyclopedia.ca/en/article/henry-morgentaler/.

Martin, M. 2000. *Meaningful Work: Rethinking Professional Ethics*. New York: Oxford University Press.

Mastromatteo, M. 2003. Alberta Pharmacist Wins Concessions in Right-to-refuse Case, *The Interim: Canada's Life and Family Newspaper*. Retrieved on June 14, 2019 athttp://www.theinterim.com/issues/alberta-pharmacist-wins-concessions-in-right-to-refuse-case/.

May, S. C. 2005. Principled Compromise and the Abortion Controversy, *Philosophy & Public Affairs* 33(4): 317–48.

May, S. C. 2015. Compromise. In the *International Encyclopedia of Ethics*. Ed. H. LaFollette. Chichester: John Wiley & Sons.

McCullough, L. B. and S. Wear. 1985. Respect for Autonomy and Medical Paternalism Reconsidered, *Theoretical Medicine* 6(3): 295–308.

McDonald, E. dir. 2008. Pregnant Man. [film] September Films.

McFall, L. 1987. Integrity, *Ethics* 98(1): 5–20.

McGeer, V. 2008. Trust, Hope, and Empowerment, *Australasian Journal of Philosophy* 86(2): 237–54.

McInerney, P. K. 1990. Does a Fetus Already Have a Future-like-ours? *Journal of Philosophy* 87(5): 264–8.

McLeod, C. 2002. *Self-Trust and Reproductive Autonomy*. Cambridge, MA: MIT Press.

McLeod, C. 2004. Integrity and Self-Protection, *Journal of Social Philosophy* 35(2): 216–32.

McLeod, C. 2005. How to Distinguish Autonomy from Integrity, *Canadian Journal of Philosophy* 35(1): 107–34.

McLeod, C. 2008. Referral in the Wake of Conscientious Objection to Abortion, *Hypatia* 23(4): 30–47.

McLeod, C. 2012. Taking a Feminist Relational Perspective on Conscience. In *Being Relational: Reflections on Relational Theory and Health Law and Policy*. Ed. J. Downie and J. Lewellyn. Vancouver: University of British Columbia Press. Pp. 161–81.

McLeod, C. 2014. The Denial of "Artificial" Contraception by Ottawa Doctors, *Impact Ethics*. Retrieved on June 13, 2019 at https://impactethics.ca/2014/03/04/the-denial-of-artificial-contraception-by-ottawa-doctors/.

McLeod, C. 2015. Trust. In the *Stanford Encyclopedia of Philosophy*. Ed. Edward N. Zalta. Originally published 2006. Retrieved on June 13, 2019 at http://plato.stanford.edu/entries/trust/.

McLeod, C. 2017. The Medical Nonnecessity of In Vitro Fertilization, *IJFAB: International Journal of Feminist Approaches to Bioethics* 10(1): 78–102.

McLeod, C. and F. Baylis. 2007. Donating Fresh vs. Frozen Embryos to Stem Cell Research: In Whose Interests? *Bioethics* 21(9): 465–77.

McLeod, C. and C. Fitzgerald. 2015. Conscientious Refusal and Access to Abortion and Contraception. In the *Routledge Companion to Bioethics*. Ed. J. Arras, E. Fenton, and R. Kukla. New York: Routledge. Pp. 343–56.

McLeod, C. and E. Ryman. 2020. Trust, Autonomy, and Fiduciaries. In *Fiduciaries and Trust: Ethics, Politics, Economics, and Law*. Ed. P. B. Miller and M. Harding. Cambridge: Cambridge University Press. Pp. 74–86.

Medical Board of Australia. 2014. Good Medical Practice: A Code of Conduct for Doctors in Australia. Retrieved June 15, 2019 at https://www.medicalboard.gov.au/documents/default.aspx?record=WD14%2f13332&dbid=AP&chksum=1GnSQD5LhB2UvesdywVfbw%3d%3d.

Merritt, P. 2008. Lesbian Refused IVF Treatment in California, *Rewire*. June 2. Retrieved on June 13, 2019 at https://rewire.news/article/2008/06/02/lesbian-refused-ivf-treatment-california/.

Meyers, C. and R. Woods. 1996. An Obligation to Provide Abortion Services: What Happens When Physicians Refuse? *Journal of Medical Ethics* 22: 115–20.

Mill, J. S. 1851/1989. *"On Liberty" and Other Writings*. Ed. S. Collini. Cambridge: Cambridge University Press.

Miller, P. 2000. Religion, Reproductive Health and Access to Services, *Conscience* 21(2): 2–8.

Miller, P. B. 2011. A Theory of Fiduciary Liability, *McGill Law Journal* 56(2): 235–88.

Miller, P. B. 2014. The Fiduciary Relationship. In *Philosophical Foundations of Fiduciary Law*. Ed. P. B. Miller and A. S. Gold. Oxford: Oxford University Press. Pp. 63–90.

Miller, P. and A. Gold. 2015. Fiduciary Governance, *William & Mary Law Review* 57(2): 513–86.

Milne, V., L. Laupacis, and M. Tierney. 2014. Are Family Doctors Cherry Picking Patients? *Healthy Debate*. Retrieved on June 13, 2019 at http://healthydebate. ca/2014/10/topic/family-doctors-cherry-picking-patients.

Mullin, A. 2005. Trust, Social Norms, and Motherhood, *Journal of Social Philosophy* 36(3): 316–30.

Murphy, J. E., R. A. Forrey, and U. Desiraju. 2004. Community Pharmacists' Responses to Drug–Drug Interaction Alerts, *American Journal of Health-System Pharmacy* 61: 1484–7.

National Association of Boards of Pharmacy. 2003. Model Pharmacy Act. Park Ridge, IL.

Norris, A., D. Bessett, J. R. Steinberg, M. L. Kavanaugh, S. De Zordo, and D. Becker. 2011. Abortion Stigma: A Reconceptualization of Constituents, Causes, and Consequences, *Women's Health Issues* 21(3): S49–54.

O'Neill, O. 2002. *Trust and Autonomy in Bioethics*. Cambridge, UK: Cambridge UP.

Ontario College of Pharmacists. 2015. Code of Ethics. Retrieved June 15, 2019 at http://www.ocpinfo.com/library/council/download/CodeofEthics2015.pdf.

Ontario College of Pharmacists. 2016. Professional Obligations When Declining to Provide a Pharmacy Product or Service Due to Conscience or Religion. Retrieved on June 14, 2019 at http://www.ocpinfo.com/regulations-standards/policies-guidelines/refusal/.

Osnos, E. 2002. NYC Leads New Effort to Train MDs in Abortions, *Chicago Tribune*, July 4. Retrieved on June 13, 2019 at http://articles.chicagotribune.com/2002-07-04/news/0207040129_1_abortion-training-abortion-providers-abortion-rights-advocates.

Peck, R., W. Rella, J. Tudela, J. Aznar, and B. Mozzanega. 2016. Does Levonorgestrel Emergency Contraceptive Have a Post-fertilization Effect? A Review of its Mechanism of Action, *The Linacre Quarterly* 83(1): 35–51.

Pellegrino, E. D. 1991. Trust and Distrust in Professional Ethics. In *Ethics, Trust and the Professions: Philosophical and Cultural Aspects*. Ed. E. D. Pellegrino, R. M. Veatch, and J. P. Langan. Washington, DC: Georgetown University Press. Pp. 69–89.

Pellegrino, E. D. 2002. The Physician's Conscience, Conscience Clauses, and Religious Belief: A Catholic Perspective, *Fordham Urban Law Journal* 30(1): 221–44.

Pellegrino, E. D. and D. C. Thomasma. 1993. *The Virtues in Medical Practice*. New York: Oxford University Press.

Pelley, L. 2015. Christian Doctors' Group Says New College Policy Infringes on Freedom of Conscience, *The Toronto Star*, March 24. Retrieved on June 13, 2019 at http://www.thestar.com/life/health_wellness/2015/03/24/christian-doctors-group-says-new-college-policy-infringes-on-freedom-of-conscience.html.

Pharmaceutical Society of Australia. 2017. Code of Ethics for Pharmacists. Retrieved June 15, 2019 at https://www.psa.org.au/wp-content/uploads/2018/07/PSA-Code-of-Ethics-2017.pdf.

Piper, A. 1990. Higher-order Discrimination. In *Identity, Character, and Morality: Essays in Moral Psychology*. Ed. O. Flanagan and A. O. Rorty. Cambridge, MA: MIT Press. Pp. 285–309.

Planned Parenthood Federation of America. 2013. Myths about Abortion and Breast Cancer. Retrieved on June 13, 2019 at: http://www.plannedparenthood.org/ files/9613/9611/5578/Myths_About_Abortion_and_Breast_Cancer.pdf.

Ploug, T. and S. Holm. 2015. Doctors, Patients, and Nudging in the Clinical Context—Four Views on Nudging and Informed Consent, *The American Journal of Bioethics* 15(10): 28–38.

Polizogopoulos, A. 2014. College of Physicians and Surgeons Ontario Policy #5-08: *Physicians and the Human Rights Code*. Submission made to the CPSO on behalf of the Christian Medical and Dental Society of Canada and the Canadian Federation of Catholic Physician Societies. Retrieved on June 13, 2019 at http:// www.cmdscanada.org/my_folders/Position_Papers/Submissions_of_the_CMDS_ and_the_CFCPS_1.pdf.

Prieur, Rev. M. 2004. Cooperation in Bioethical Wrongdoing: When Should a Believer Get Out of the Game? Unpublished manuscript. Presented at King's University College, London ON.

Quigley, M. 2013. Nudging for Health: On Public Policy and Designing Choice Architecture, *Medical Law Review* 21(4): 588–621.

Quill, T. E. and H. Brody. 1996. Physician Recommendations and Patient Autonomy: Finding a Balance between Physician Power and Patient Choice, *Annals of Internal Medicine* 125(9): 763–8.

Rafie, S., R. H. Stone, T. A. Wilkinson, L. M. Borgelt, S. Y. El-Ibiary, and D. Ragland. 2017. Role of the Community Pharmacist in Emergency Contraception Counseling and Delivery in the United States: Current Trends and Future Prospects, *Integrated Pharmacy Research and Practice* 6: 99–108.

Rawls, J. 1971. *A Theory of Justice*. Cambridge, MA: Harvard University Press.

Raz, J. 1986. *The Morality of Freedom*. Oxford: Clarendon Press.

Roberts, D. 1997. *Killing the Black Body: Race, Reproduction, and the Meaning of Liberty*. New York: Vintage.

Robinson, B. 1997. Birds Do It. Bees Do It. So Why Not Single Women and Lesbians? *Bioethics* 11: 217–27.

Rodrigues, S. 2014. A Woman's Right to Know? Forced Ultrasound Measures as an Intervention of Biopower, *IJFAB: International Journal of Feminist Approaches to Bioethics* 7(1): 51–73.

Rodwin, M. A. 1995. Strains in the Fiduciary Metaphor: Divided Physician Loyalties and Obligations in a Changing Health Care System, *American Journal of Law and Medicine* 21(2–3): 241–57.

Rowland, D. 2004. *The Boundaries of her Body: The Troubling History of Women's Rights in America*. Naperville, IL: Sphinx.

Ryle, G. 1940. Conscience and Moral Convictions, *Analysis* 7: 31–9.

Ryman, E. 2017. Fiduciary Duties and Commercial Surrogacy. PhD Dissertation. Western University. Retrieved June 13, 2019 at http://ir.lib.uwo.ca/etd/4728/.

Saltzman, L. E., C. H. Johnson, B. C. Gilbert, and M. M. Goodwin. 2003. Physical Abuse around the Time of Pregnancy: An Examination of Prevalence and Risk Factors in 16 States, *Maternal and Child Health Journal* 7(1): 31–43.

Samet, I. 2008. Guarding the Fiduciary's Conscience—A Justification of a Stringent Profit-stripping Rule, *Oxford Journal of Legal Studies* 28(4): 763–81.

Sample, R. 2003. *Exploitation: What It Is and Why It's Wrong*. Lanham, MD: Rowman & Littlefield.

Sanger-Katz, M. 2019. Trump Administration Strengthens "Conscience Rule" for Health Care Workers, *New York Times*, May 2. Retrieved on June 14, 2019 at https://www.nytimes.com/2019/05/02/upshot/conscience-rule-trump-religious-exemption-health-care.html.

Savulescu, J. 2006. Conscientious Objection in Medicine, *BMJ* 332(2).

Savulescu, J. and U. Schuklenk. 2017. Doctors Have No Right to Refuse Medical Assistance in Dying, Abortion, or Contraception, *Bioethics* 31(3):162–70.

Schuklenk, U. 2015. Conscientious Objection in Medicine: Private Ideological Convictions Must Not Supersede Public Service Obligations, *Bioethics* 29: ii–iii.

Schuklenk, U. and R. Smalling. 2016. Why Medical Professionals Have No Moral Claim to Conscientious Objection Accommodation in Liberal Democracies, *Journal of Medical Ethics* 43(4): 234–40.

Schulz, M., R. Goebel, C. Schumann, and P. Zagermann-Muncke. 2016. Non-prescription Dispensing of Emergency Oral Contraceptives: Recommendations from the German Federal Chamber of Pharmacists [Bundesapothekerkammer], *Pharmacy Practice* 14(3): 828.

Sciaraffa, S. 2009. Identification, Meaning, and the Normativity of Social Roles, *European Journal of Philosophy* 19(1): 107–28.

Shadd, P. and J. Shadd. 2017. Institutional Non-participation in Assisted Dying: Changing the Conversation, *Bioethics* 33: 207–14.

Shaw, J. 2006. Reality Check: A Close Look at Accessing Abortion Services in Canadian Hospitals. Ottawa: Canadians for Choice.

Shaw, J. 2013. Abortion as a Social Justice Issue in Contemporary Canada, *Critical Social Work* 14(2). Retrieved on June 13, 2019 at http://www1.uwindsor.ca/criticalsocialwork/abortion_in_canada.

Sherwin, S. 1998. A Relational Approach to Autonomy in Health Care. In *The Politics of Women's Health: Exploring Agency and Autonomy*. Ed. The Feminist Health Care Ethics Research Network. Temple University Press. Pp. 19–47.

Shoveller, J., C. Chabot, J. A. Soon, and M. Levine. 2007. Identifying Barriers to Emergency Contraception Use among Young Women from Various Sociocultural Groups in British Columbia, Canada, *Perspectives on Sexual and Reproductive Health* 39(1): 13–20.

Smith, M. 2008. Terrorism, Shared Rules, and Trust, *Journal of Political Philosophy* 16(2): 201–19.

Smith, L. 2014. Fiduciary Relationships: Ensuring the Loyal Exercise of Judgement on Behalf of Another, *The Law Quarterly Review* 130(Oct): 608–34.

Stein, R. 2005. Pharmacists' Rights at Front of New Debate, *Washington Post* March 28: A01.

Stein, R. 2006. A Medical Crisis of Conscience: Faith Drives Some to Refuse Patients Medication or Care, *Washington Post* Sunday, July 16: A01.

Stoljar, D. 2009. The Argument from Revelation. In *Conceptual Analysis and Philosophical Naturalism*. Ed. D. Braddon-Mitchell and R. Nola. Cambridge, MA: MIT Press. Pp. 113–37.

Stoljar, N. 2011. Different Women: Gender and the Realism-Nominalism Debate. In *Feminist Metaphysics: Explorations in the Ontology of Sex, Gender and the Self*. Ed. C. Witt. New York: Springer. Pp. 27–46.

Sulmasy, D. 2008. What Is Conscience and Why Is Respect for It So Important? *Theoretical Medicine and Bioethics* 29(3): 135–49.

Tannenbaum, C. and N. L. Sheehan. 2014. Understanding and Preventing Drug–Drug and Drug–Gene Interactions, *Expert Review of Clinical Pharmacology* 7(4): 533–44.

Taylor, G. 1987. *Pride, Shame, and Guilt: Emotions of Self-Assessment*. New York: Oxford University Press.

Thaler, R. H, and C. R. Sunstein. 2008. *Nudge: Improving Decisions about Health, Wealth, and Happiness*. New Haven, CT: Yale University Press.

Thomson, J. J. 1971. A Defense of Abortion, *Philosophy & Public Affairs* 1(1): 47–66.

Thomson, J. J. 1986. Feinberg on Harm, Offense, and the Criminal Law: A Review Essay, *Philosophy & Public Affairs* 15(4): 381–95.

Tweedy, D. 2015. The Case for Black Doctors, *The New York Times*, May 15. Retrieved on June 13, 2019 at: http://www.nytimes.com/2015/05/17/opinion/sunday/the-case-for-black-doctors.html?_r=0.

van Bogaert, L.-J. 2002. The Limits of Conscientious Objection to Abortion in the Developing World, *Developing World Bioethics* 2(2): 131–43.

Veatch, R. M. 1991. *The Patient-Physician Relation: The Patient as Partner, Part 2*. Bloomington: Indiana University Press.

Veatch, R. M. 1999. The Pharmacist and Assisted Suicide, *American Journal of Health-System Pharmacy* 56: 260–6.

Vischer, R. K. 2006. Conscience in Context: Pharmacist Rights and the Eroding Moral Marketplace, *Stanford Law and Policy Review* 17: 83–119.

Walker, M. U. 1998. *Moral Understandings: A Feminist Study in Ethics*. New York: Routledge.

Walker, M. U. 2006. Damages to Trust. In her *Moral Repair: Reconstructing Moral Relations after Wrongdoing*. Cambridge: Cambridge University Press. Pp. 72–109.

Wall, L. L. and D. Brown. 2006. Refusals by Pharmacists to Dispense Emergency Contraception: A Critique, *Obstetrics and Gynecology* 107(5): 1148–51.

Weitz, A. W., K. Moore, R. Gordon, and N. Adler. 2008. You Say "Regret" and I Say "Relief": A Need to Break the Polemic about Abortion, *Contraception* 78: 87–9.

Weitz, T., D. Taylor, S. Desai, U. D. Upadhyay, J. Waldman, M. F. Battistelli, and E. A. Drey. 2013. Safety of Aspiration Abortion Performed by Nurse Practitioners, Certified Nurse Midwives, and Physician Assistants under a California Legal Waiver, *American Journal of Public Health* 103(3): 454–61.

Whitbeck, C. 1983. The Moral Implications of Regarding Women as People: New Perspectives on Pregnancy and Personhood. In *Abortion and the Status of the Fetus*. Ed. W. Bondeson et al. Dordrecht: Reidel. Pp. 242–72.

Whitbeck, C. 1995. Trust. In *The Encyclopedia of Bioethics*. 2nd ed. New York: MacMillan.

Wicclair, M. R. 2000. Conscientious Objection in Medicine, *Bioethics* 14: 205–27.

Wicclair, M. R. 2006. Pharmacies, Pharmacists, and Conscientious Objection, *Kennedy Institute of Ethics Journal* 16(3): 225–50.

Wicclair, M. R. 2011. *Conscientious Objection in Health Care: An Ethical Analysis.* Cambridge: Cambridge University Press.

Wicclair, M. R. 2017. Conscientious Objection in Healthcare and Moral Integrity, *Cambridge Quarterly of Healthcare Ethics* 26: 7–17.

Wiedenmayer, K., R. S. Summers, C. A. Mackie, A. G. S. Gous, and M. Everard. 2006. Developing Pharmacy Practice: A Focus on Patient Care. World Health Organization and the International Pharmaceutical Federation. Retrieved June 14, 2019 at https://apps.who.int/iris/handle/10665/69399.

World Health Organization. 2015. Health Workers' Roles in Providing Safe Abortion Care and Post-abortion Contraception. Retrieved June 14, 2019 at https://www.who.int/reproductivehealth/publications/unsafe_abortion/abortion-task-shifting/en/.

Worthen, L. 2014. Letter on Behalf of the Christian Medical and Dental Society of Canada and the Canadian Federation of Catholic Physician Societies to the College of Physicians and Surgeons of Ontario about Its Draft Policy, *Physicians and the Human Rights Code.* Retrieved on June 13, 2019 at http://www.cmdscanada.org/my_folders/Position_Papers/Letter_to_CPSO_August_5_2014.pdf.

Wu, J., T. Gipson, N. Chin, L. L. Wynn, K. Cleland, C. Morrison, and J. Trussell. 2007. Women Seeking Emergency Contraceptive Pills by Using the Internet, *Obstetrics & Gynecology* 110(1): 44–52.

Zaner, R. 1991. The Phenomenon of Trust and the Patient–Physician Relationship. In *Ethics, Trust, and the Professions.* Ed. E. D. Pellegrino, R. M. Veatch, and J. P. Langan. Washington, DC: Georgetown University Press. Pp. 45–67.

Ziskin, L., and I. Bryce. 2002. Spider-Man. [film] Columbia Pictures et al.

Zwolinski, M. and A. Wertheimer. 2016. Exploitation. In the *Stanford Encyclopedia of Philosophy.* Ed. E. Zalta. Retrieved on Nov. 10, 2019 at https://plato.stanford.edu/entries/exploitation/.

Index